Zainab Anber

Effect of Diazepam on steroidogenesis and spermatogenesis in male rats

Zainab Anber

Effect of Diazepam on steroidogenesis and spermatogenesis in male rats

Noor Publishing

Imprint
Any brand names and product names mentioned in this book are subject to trademark, brand or patent protection and are trademarks or registered trademarks of their respective holders. The use of brand names, product names, common names, trade names, product descriptions etc. even without a particular marking in this work is in no way to be construed to mean that such names may be regarded as unrestricted in respect of trademark and brand protection legislation and could thus be used by anyone.

Cover image: www.ingimage.com

Publisher:
Noor Publishing
is a trademark of
International Book Market Service Ltd., member of OmniScriptum Publishing Group
17 Meldrum Street, Beau Bassin 71504, Mauritius

Printed at: see last page
ISBN: 978-620-2-35049-5

Copyright © Zainab Anber
Copyright © 2018 International Book Market Service Ltd., member of OmniScriptum Publishing Group

Dedication

To

My

Family

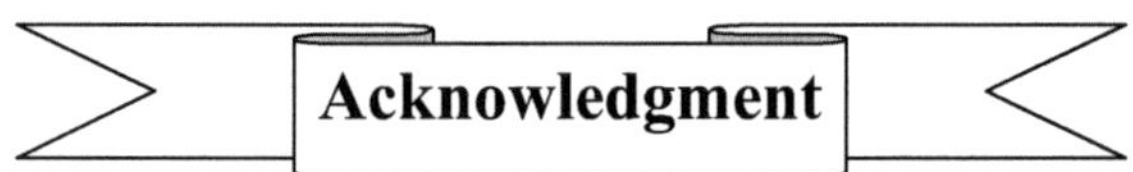

Acknowledgment

Praise is to our almighty gracious Allah for enabling me to finish and present this work.

I would like to express my heartfelt gratitude and appreciation to my supervisor Prof. Dr. **Mohammed A. Taher**, for his scientific guidance, valuable advice, generosity, help and encouragement throughout the course of this work.

My profound and sincere thanks expressed to Dr. **Salim Al-Obaidy** for his assistance in the histopathology analysis with extreme gratefulness.

Finally, I would like to express my deep gratitude to all kind, helpful and lovely people who helped directly or indirectly to complete this work.

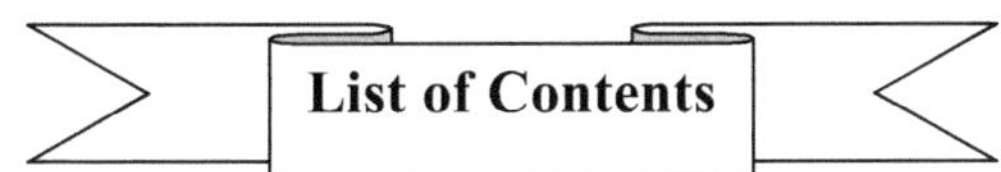

List of Contents

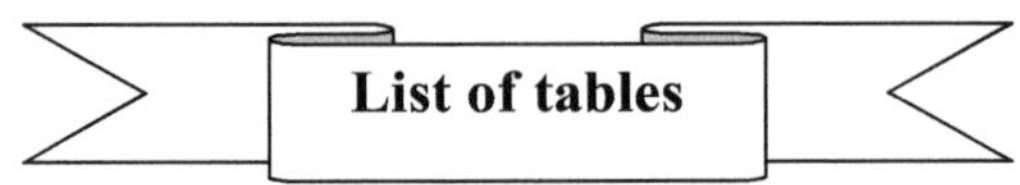

List of tables

Table no.	Title
2-1	List of the drugs used with their companies
2-2	List of chemicals with their suppliers
2-3	List of kits with their suppliers
2-4	List of instruments with their suppliers
2-5	Conditions for conversion of RNA into cDNA
2-6	Conditions for real-time PCR
2-7	Primer sequence for the StAR gene
2-8	Primer sequence for the ß-actin gene
3-1	The effect of different oral doses of diazepam suspension and sulfasalazine on the testicular, epididymis, seminal vesicle and prostate gland weight to body weight ratio in male rats.
3-2	Effect of different oral doses of diazepam suspension and sulfasalazine on the sperm characteristics of male rats
3-3	Effect of different oral doses of diazepam suspension on the grades of motility in male rats
3-4	Effect of different oral doses of diazepam suspension on the serum levels of hormones in male rats
3-5	Effect of different oral doses of diazepam suspension on the fertility index
3-6	Relative gene expression between groups using RT-qPCR

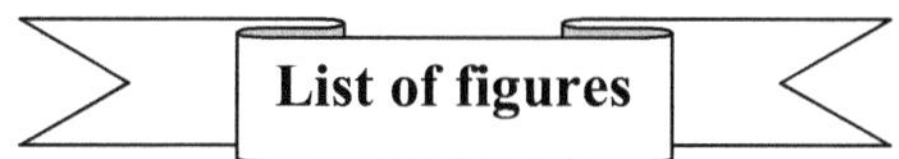

List of figures

A260/A 280	Absorbance at 260 and 280 nm
ANOVA	Analysis of variance
B.W.	Body weight
Ca^{+2}	Calcium
cDNA	Complementary deoxy ribonucleic acid
Ct	Cycle threshold
CYP	Cytochrome p450
CYP11A	Cytochrome p450 family 11, subfamily A
DAG	Di acyl Glycerol
DEPC	Diethylpyrocarbonate
DNA	Deoxyribonucleic acid
EDTA	Ethylene diamine tetra acetic acid
ELISA	Enzyme-linked immunosorbent assay
FSH	Follicle stimulating hormone
GABA A	Gama amino butyric acid type A
GnRH	Gonadotropin Releasing Hormone
GnRHR	Gonadotropin Releasing Hormone Receptor
GR	Glutathione reductase
H&E	Hematoxylin and Eosin
hcG	Human chorionic gonadotropin
HDL	High density lipoprotein
HH	hypogonadotropic hypogonadism
HRP	Horseradish peroxidase
IH	Inhibin hormone
IM	Intramuscularly
IP3	Inositol tri phosphate
IV	Intravenously
KDa	Kilo Dalton
LD50	Lethal dose 50%
LDL	Low density lipoprotein
LH	Luteinizing Hormone
LHß	Luteinizing Hormone subunit beta
mIU	Miliinternational unit
mRNA	Messenger ribonucleic acid

Na$^+$	Sodium ion
O.D	Optical density
PBR	Peripheral benzodiazepine receptor
PCR	Polymerase chain reaction
PGA	Pituitary- gonadal axis
4-PL	four parameter logestic
qPCR	Quantitative (real-time) polymerase chain reaction
PIP2	Phosphatidyl Insitol Dihphophate
PLC	Phospho Lipase C
RBC	Red blood cell
RNA	Ribonucleic acid
Rpm	Rotation per minute
RT-PCR	Reverse transcription polymerase chain reaction
SE	Standard error
SOD	Superoxide dismutase
SPSS	Statistical package for social sciences
StAR	Steroidogenic acute regulatory protein
TM	Trade mark
TSPO	Translocator protein
UV	Ultraviolet
VDCCs	Voltage dependent calcium channels
VLDL	Very low density lipoprotein
Wt.	weight

Abstract

Background

Infertility is one of the most serious problems around the world and the male counterpart contributes half of the infertility cases. Infertility can be caused by androgen deficiency or low testosterone level. The evaluation of infertility can aid in determining the underlying cause of infertility as well as giving treatment to allow conception to occur. Diazepam is used to treat anxiety, convulsions, myorelaxation and for sedation . The severity of adverse effects induced by diazepam forces physicians to pay attention and exercise caution to side effects when they prescribe this drug. Recent studies found that diazepam acts as Ca^{+2} channels antagonist as it can produce a complete inhibition of voltage-dependent Ca^{+2} uptake and that the Na^{+}/Ca^{+2} exchange carrier in mitochondria may be a common receptor for diazepam and calcium channel blockers. The endocrine control of Leydig cell steroidogenic activity by follicle stimulating hormone or luteinizing hormone (LH)   has been exerted through their respective receptors coupled to the Ca^{2+}mediated signaling pathway . Calcium ion contributes in many cellular functions in both somatic and germ cells in the testis, especially, mediating the responses to endocrine hormones and local regulators in genital tracts and thus any change in the transport of Ca^{+2} across the cell membrane could result in an extreme impact on steroidogenesis and spermatogenesis .

Objective

The aim of this study was to investigate whether treatment of male rats with diazepam interferes with the fertility status, especially the effects of diazepam on steroidogenesis and spermatogenesis.

Materials and methods

Fifty male rats (200-250) gm were divided into five groups; control group (n=10) and test groups that received (2, 5and 10mg/kg/day) of diazepam by oral gavage, each one (n=10) and sulfasalazine (500mg/kg/day) for 8 weeks. Animals were kept in standard conditions. At the last day of experiment, animals were weighed, sacrificed and the testes, epididymis, seminal vesicles and prostate were removed and weighed. Sperms were collected from the epididymis and the sperm concentration, motility, viability and morplological abnormalities were examined. Serum LH, FSH and testosterone were measured using rat ELISA kits. Also the fertility index was examined. Histological sections were also taken for both the testis and epididymis. In addition, the effects of diazepam on the testicular steroidogenic acute regulatory protein (StAR) mRNA expression were determined by using reverse transcription – polymerase chain reaction analysis.

Results

The results of the present study showed that treatment with diazepam in a dose-dependent pattern (2, 5 and 10 mg/kg/day)   highly significantly ($P<0.001$) decrease the mean testes, epididymis, seminal vesicles and prostate weight to the body weight ratio. Sperm concentration, motility and viability were highly significantly ($P<0.001$) decreased .Also, the morphologically abnormal sperms percentage were highly significantly ($P<0.001$) increased. Different effects of the drug were recorded on the four grades of sperm motility;   mainly a significant ($P<0.05$) decrease in the progressive and curve motility and a significant ($P<0.05$) increase in the insitu and the immotile percentage with increasing the dose of the drug. Serum LH, FSH and testosterone levels were highly significantly ($P<0.001$) decreased. The fertility index examination showed a significant ($p<0.05$) decrease. Histological sections showed structural changes in the testes like loss of some of the spermatogenesis stages and decrease in number of sertoli and Leydig cells with increasing the dose of diazepam with a corresponding decrease in the number of sperms in both the testes and epididymis. Diazepam treatment also inhibit the (StAR) mRNA relative gene expression in testes and had a greater effect at dose (10 mg/kg/day) that is highly significantly ($P<0.001$) decreased compared to that produced by other doses of the drug.

Conclusion

Diazepam, in a dose –dependent pattern, was effective in causing a significant arrest of developing spermatids and diminishing steroidogenesis by abrogating StAR protein gene expression in rats testes.

Chapter one

Male infertility

1.1 Definition

Male infertility refers to the inability of a male to achieve pregnancy in a fertile female. It is estimated that 60% of married couples having regular unprotected intercourse, achieve pregnancy after 6 months of co-habitation, 90% achieve pregnancy by 12 months and 95% between18-24 months [1].   Recently, infertility is defined as failure to conceive after regular unprotected sexual intercourse for 2 years in the absence of known reproductive pathology [2].

1.2 Etiology

The causes of male infertility can be divided into four main areas:

1. Hypothalamic-pituitary disease 1-2%.
2. Primary hypogonadism 30-40%.
3. Disorders of sperm transport 10-20%.
4. Idiopathic 40-50% [3].

1.2.1 Hypothalamic-Pituitary (pre-testicular) disease

Any hypothalamic or pituitary disease can cause gonadotropin-releasing hormone (GnRH) or gonadotropin (LH and FSH) deficiency , which leads to deficiency in androgen secretion, deficiency in spermatogenesis and therefore infertility. These conditions are congenital which includes Kallmann syndrome, genetic disorders, pituitary and hypothalamic tumors, hormonal and medications, acquired as in trauma or systemic disorders as in chronic illness, nutrition and obesity [4].

1.2.2 Primary hypogonadism (testicular) disease

Primary gonadal deficiency is an important cause of azospermia and oligospermia. Congenital or developmental disorders, disorders of androgen receptor, Y chromosome defect, and acquired disorders such as infection, drugs, environmental toxins, and smoking can cause infertility [5].

1.2.3 Disorders of sperm transport (Post-testicular) disease

Often called obstructive azospermia is due to either dysfunction in ejaculation or the sperm delivery is obstructed. The obstruction comes from the vas deferens, epididymis, or ejaculatory duct and can be congenital or acquired [6].

1.2.4 Idiopathic infertility

No reason related to male infertility can be identified i.e, unremarkable physical examination, no history of infertility and endocrine laboratory evaluation is normal. Idiopathic male infertility may be due to disruption in the endocrine system due to pollution of environment, oxidative stress or genetic abnormalities [7].

1.3 The male reproductive system

The male reproductive system comprises the testes, epididymis, vas deferens, accessory sex glands and penis which together produce and transfer the ejaculate which comprises spermatozoa and seminal fluid [8].

1.3.1 Testes

The testes are the main male reproductive glands and they are considered as mixed glands; have two main functions: act as exocrine glands through production of spermatozoa in seminiferous tubules, and act as endocrine glands by production of androgens from Leydig cells [9].

Histologically, the testis are covered by dense fibrous connective tissue known as Tunica albuginea which is covered by a layer of connective tissue rich with blood vessels, called Tunica vaginalis; there are some bounds originated from Tunica albuginea, which divide testes into many lobules and these bounds are fused with each other again and form a structure of connective tissue called Mediastinum testis [10].

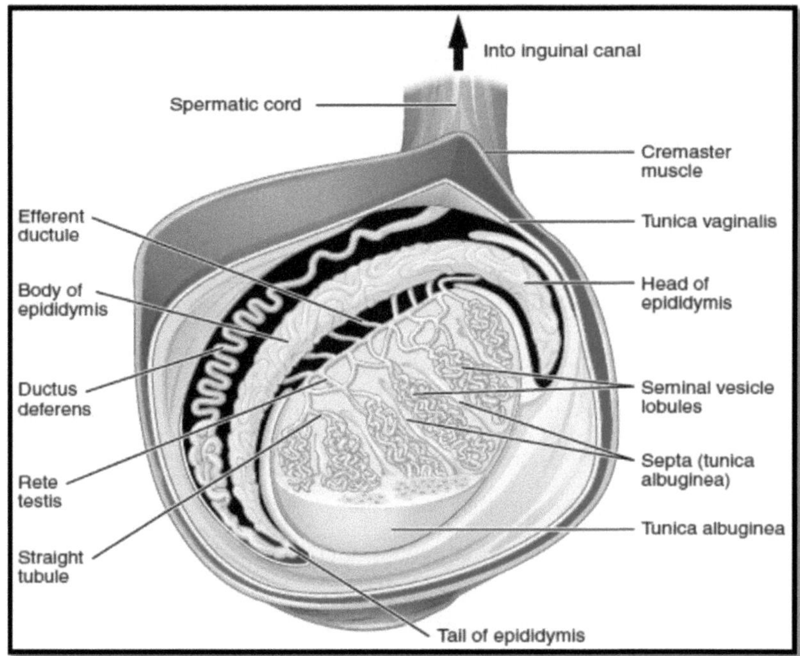

Figure (1-1) Structure of the male testes [11]

Functionally, the testis has three parts: the interstitial tissue containing the Leydig cells surrounding the seminiferous tubules which bathe them with testosterone rich fluid. The other two parts reside within seminiferous tubules, the basal part contains spermatogonia which is divided through mitosis, where as the ad luminal represents a good environment for spermatocytes to be converted into spermatid and then into spermatozoa through meiosis. Within the seminiferous tubules, the

Sertoli cells, which extend from the basal part into the ad luminal provide support and nourishment to the developing germ cells [12].

The Sertoli cells play a major role in regulation of spermatogenesis and altering rates of spermatozoa produced. Sertoli cells functions include providing structural support and nutrition to develop germ cells, phagocytosis of degenerating germ cells and residual bodies, release of spermatid at spermiation and production of a host of proteins that regulate or respond to pituitary hormone release and that influence mitotic activity of spermatogonia [13].

1.3.2 Epididymis

The epididymis is a male accessory organ located between the efferent ducts and the vas deferens, characterized by a single coiled tubule duct.The anatomic segments of the epididymis include the initial segment, the caput, the corpus and the cauda. Each region consists of a lumen and an epithelium composed mostly of principle and basal cells [14]. The epididymal duct is now recognized as a channel that transports, concentrates and stores the spermatozoa. It is also known that the spermatozoa leaving the testis are immovable, immature and unable to fertilize an oocyte [15], and that under androgen control, the epididymal epithelium secretes proteins within the intraluminal compartment that create a very complex environment surrounding the spermatozoa [16]. The epididymal duct produces the morphological, biochemical, physiological and functional changes to the structures of the spermatozoa through a process known as epididymal maturation which converts the spermatozoa into fertilization – competent cells [17].

1.3.3 Vas deferens

The ductus (vas) deferens also called sperm duct or spermatic deferens extends from the epididymis in the scrotum on its own side into the abdominal cavity through the inguinal canal. The inguinal canal is an opening in the abdominal wall for the spermatic cord, a connective tissue sheath that contains the ductus deferens, testicular blood vessels and nerves. The smooth muscle layer of the ductus deferens contracts in waves of peristalsis during ejaculation [18].

1.3.4 The accessory male glands

The main male accessory male glands include the seminal vesicle, prostate gland, and bulbourethral glands. These glands secrete fluid into the semen; each fluid with different biochemical characteristics. While the seminiferous tubules and the epididymis compose only about 5% of the volume of semen. The main functions of these glands is to activate the spermatozoa, provide nutrients for sperm motility, propel the spermatozoa and fluids mixture through the reproductive tract by peristaltic movement and to produce buffers that counteract the acidity of urethral and vaginal contents [19].

1.4 Spermatogenesis

Spermatogenesis is the total process which takes place in the semniferous tubules started from spermatogonia and finished by production of spermatozoa [20]. Spermatogenesis is a continuous process to produce a great number of spermatozoa throughout life [21]. The spermatogenesis process starts from spermatogonia stem cells in the basement membrane of the seminiferous tubules that proliferate and differentiate into primary spermatocytes, secondary spermatocytes, spermatids and spermatozoa [22], figure (1-2).

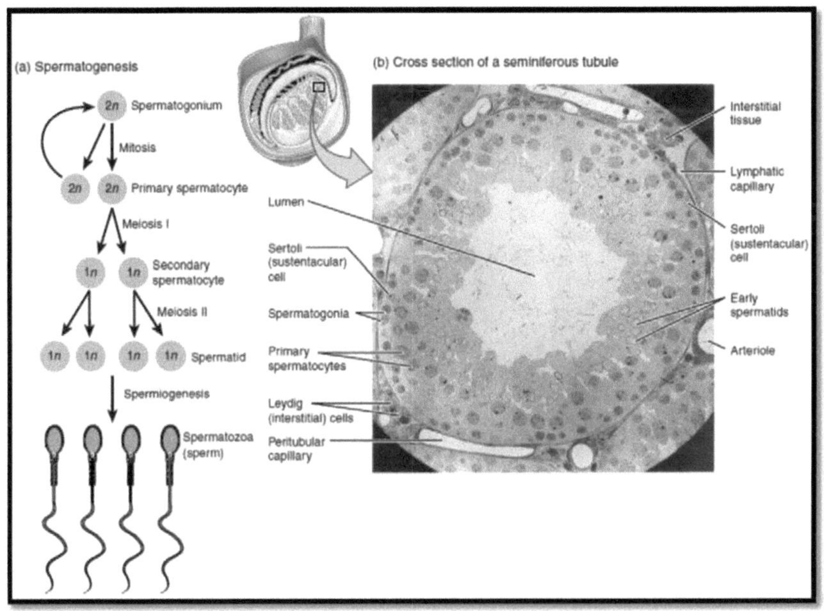

Figure (1-2) The process of spermatogenesis [23].

The overall duration of spermatogenesis is calculated as 51-56 days in rats, 37-43 days in different monkey species, 35 days in mice, and at least 64 days in man [24, 25,26].

1.4.1 Hormonal regulation of spermatogenesis

The spermatogenesis process takes place under hormonal control by an axis called Hypothalamic-Pitutary-Testicular axis; this axis acts by some hormones that regulate spermatogenesis in mammals. The hypothalamus releases the gonadotropin releasing hormone (GnRH) which stimulates the pituitary gland to release the follicle stimulating hormone (FSH) and lutenizing hormone (LH) [27]. The FSH stimulates sertoli cells to produce Inhibin hormone (IH) which in turn, specifically inhibits FSH secretion [28]. The LH binds to the receptors of Leydig cells which are situated in the interstitial tissue. The lutenizing hormone stimulation of Leydig cells causes the production of testosterone which is the major hormone supporting adult spermatogenesis. Although the precise function of FSH and testosterone remains elusive, the existing evidence suggest that both hormones are able to stimulate all phases of spermatogenesis. In the male FSH is required for the determination of Sertoli cell number, and for induction and maintenance of normal sperm production [29].

1.4.2 Testosterone hormone

Testosterone is the male hormone synthesized by Leydig cells of testes from cholesterol; chemically it consists of (19) carbon atom with (OH) group on the 17th carbon atom [30]. Testosterone is necessary for development and divisions of spermatogonia and increases the diameters of seminiferous tubules and acting on male reproductive system and accessory sex glands such as prostate gland, seminal vesicles and Cowpers glands by various ways [31, 32]. Additionally, testosterone is important in early embryonic stages for differentiation of Wolffian duct into epididymis and seminal vesicle; the conversion of testosterone hormone into dihydrotestosterone by 5- alpha reductase is required for masculinization of the male´s external genitalia. [33]

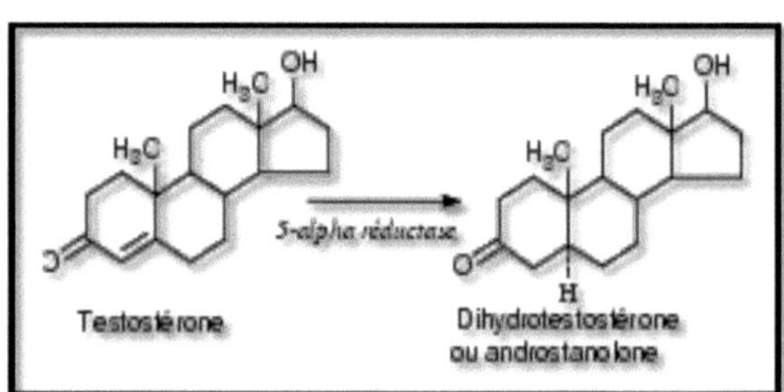

Figure(1-3) transformation of testosterone into dihydrotestosterone [33]

1.5 Diazepam

Diazepam is a benzodiazepine derivative used to treat anxiety, seizures, muscle spasm, insomnia, panic attacks, alcohol withdrawal syndrome and restless legs syndrome [34]. It possesses hypnotic, sedative, anxiolytic, anticonvulsant, skeletal muscle relaxant and amnestic properties [35].

1.5.1 Physical and chemical properties

The British Pharmacopoeia listed diazepam as a solid white or yellow crystals, it's melting point is (131.5 - 134.5)°C. It has a slightly bitter taste and it is odorless. It is documented as being very slightly soluble in water, soluble in alcohol, and freely soluble in chloroform. The pH of diazepam is neutral (i.e., pH = 7). Diazepam has a shelf life of five years for oral tablets and three years for IV/IM solutions. Diazepam should be stored at room temperature (15–30°C). The solution for parenteral injection should be protected from light and kept from freezing. The oral forms should be stored in air-tight containers and protected from light [36].

1.5.2 Chemical structure:

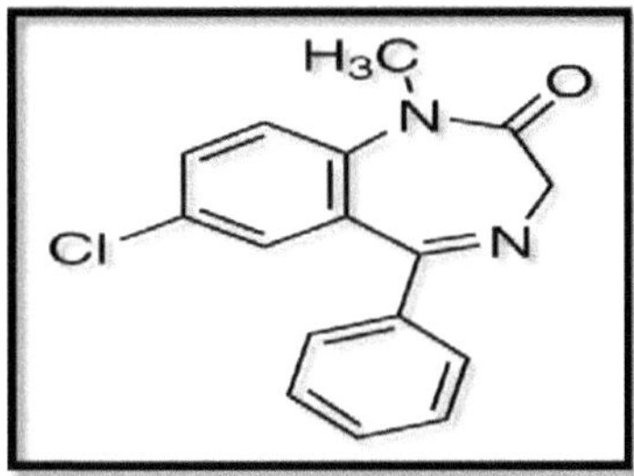

Figure (1-4) Structure of diazepam [37]

7-chloro-1 methyl-5-phenyl-3H-1,4-benzodiazepin-2-one(diazepam)

1.5.3 Mechanism of action

Diazepam acts on the GABA type A receptors ($GABA_A$). The $GABA_A$ receptors are channels selective for chloride ions activated by GABA which is the major inhibitory neurotransmitter in the brain. Binding of GABA is enhanced by benzodiazepines resulting in a greater entrance of chloride ions which in turn hyperpolarizes the cells making it very difficult to be depolarized and then the neuronal excitability is reduced [38].

1.5.4 Pharmacokinetics

Diazepam can be administered orally, intravenously (IV) intramuscularly (IM), or rectally. When administered orally, it is rapidly absorbed and has a fast onset of action. The onset of action is 1-5 minutes for IV administration and 15–30 minutes for IM administration. The duration of diazepam's peak pharmacological effects is 15 minutes to one hour for both routes of administration. Peak plasma levels occur between 30 and 90 minutes after oral administration and between 30 and 60 minutes after intramuscular administration; after rectal administration, peak plasma levels occur after 10 to 45 minutes. Diazepam is highly protein-bound, with 96 to 99% of the absorbed drug being protein-bound. The distribution half-life of diazepam is 2- 13 minutes [39].

Diazepam is highly lipid-soluble, and is widely distributed throughout the body after administration. It easily crosses both the blood–brain barrier and the placenta, and is excreted into breast milk. After absorption, diazepam is redistributed into muscle and adipose tissue. Continual daily doses of diazepam quickly build to a high concentration in the body (mainly in adipose tissue), far in excess of the actual dose for any given day [40].

Diazepam undergoes oxidative metabolism by demethylation (CYP 2C9, 2C19, 2B6, 3A4, and 3A5), hydroxylation (CYP 3A4 and 2C19) and glucuronidation in the liver. It has several pharmacologically active metabolites. The main active metabolite of diazepam is desmethyldiazepam (also known as nordazepam or nordiazepam). Its other active metabolites include the minor active metabolites temazepam and oxazepam. These metabolites are conjugated with glucuronide, and are excreted primarily in the urine. Most of the drug is metabolised; very little diazepam is excreted unchanged. The elderly metabolise benzodiazepines much more slowly than younger adults, and are also more sensitive to the effects of benzodiazepines even at similar blood plasma levels. Doses of diazepam are recommended to be about half of those given to younger people [41].

Toxicity: In adults there is no specific dose associated with death. In the few documented fatal cases, the doses have not been known with certainty and other factors complicated the clinical presentation [42].

Relevant animal data:

LD50 (oral) rat 1200 mg/kg

LD50 (oral) dog 1000 mg/kg

LD50 (oral) mice 700 mg/kg [43].

1.5.5 Adverse effects

The most common side-effects of diazepam are related to their sedating and muscle-relaxing action. They include drowsiness, dizziness, and decreased alertness and concentration. Lack of coordination may result in falls and injuries, in particular, in the elderly [44]. Another result is impairment of driving skills and increased likelihood of road traffic accidents. Decreased libido and erection problems are a common side effect. Depression and disinhibition may emerge. Hypotension and suppressed breathing (hypoventilation) may be encountered with intravenous use. Less common side effects include nausea and changes in appetite, blurred vision, confusion, euphoria, depersonalization and nightmares. Cases of liver toxicity have been described but are very rare [45,46].

1.6 Sulfasalazine

Sulfasalazine is a drug commonly used for the treatment of inflammatory bowel diseases such as ulcerative colitis and Crohn's disease. It consists of sulphapyridine linked to 5-aminosalicylic acid by an azo bond. 5-aminosalicylic acid is the active therapeutic moiety of sulfasalazine, while the most adverse effects are related to sulphapyridine. One of those is Sulfasalazine induced male infertility [47].

1.6.1 Mechanism of action

There are various mechanisms through which sulfasalazine could affect the adult reproductive system. Previous studies reported that sulfasalazine induces oxidative stress, which in turn might act as a possible mechanism of male induced infertility. Sulfasalazine induced a significant decrease of superoxide dismutase (SOD) and glutathione reductase (GR) in both testes and epididymis. Also, an increase in thiobarbituric acid-reactive substances was noted [48].

1.7 Role of Ca^{+2} ions in steroidogenesis

Calcium is one of the elements that participate in signal transduction in cells. Calcium helps regulate many cellular functions in different cells, including somatic and germ cells in the testis, as well as spermatozoa, in response to endocrine hormones and local regulators [49 - 53]. Moreover, alteration of the Ca^{2+} signaling pathway has an extreme impact on many cellular physiologies [54 -57]. Previous studies have focused on calcium channel blockers as a promising target for male contraceptive development since impaired calcium signaling is a common factor of male infertility [58]. Calcium is renewed from two Ca^{2+} sources: intracellular Ca^{2+} storage in both the endoplasmic reticulum and the mitochondria and extracellular Ca^{2+}. The extracellular Ca^{2+} must enter the cell through Ca^{2+} channels in the cell membrane before producing an effect [59]. Although an increase in Ca^{2+} is essential for the onset of Leydig cell steroidogenesis, a similar pathway for Ca^{2+} entry remains difficult to find. Some studies have suggested that cytosolic Ca^{2+} changes may result only from intracellular Ca^{2+} release [60 - 62] while other studies have argued that voltage-dependent Ca^{2+} channels (VDCCs) are also involved [63- 65]. The interaction of egg and sperm is organized around several Ca^{2+} processes include capacitation [66], acrosome reaction [67], motility [68] and hyperactivity [69].

1.8 Diazepam as calcium channel blocker

Matlib *et al.* (1983) noticed that diazepam effectively inhibit Na^+ induced Ca^{2+} release from mitochondria isolated from rabbit heart and rat brain, he suggested that the Na^+/Ca^{2+} exchange carrier in mitochondria may be a common receptor for diazepam and diltiazem (a calcium channel blocker) [70]

William *et al.* (1984) found that benzodiazepines can produce a complete inhibition of voltage-dependent Ca^{2+} uptake. Also, they indicate that benzodiazepines are acting as Ca^{2+} channels antagonists [71]. Previous studies indicated that the ability of non-neuronal type benzodiazepines to bind to a site that also binds calcium channel blocker may provide an explanation for the apparent calcium antagonist activity of the benzodiazepines in various systems. As well as for previously unexplained reports of systemic and coronary vasodilation by diazepam [72-74].

Also, Schaufele *et al.* (1995) found that diazepam relaxes the mouse urinary bladder smooth muscles; they noticed that the inhibitory effect of diazepam was similar to that induced by nifedipine (a calcium channel antagonist). They reinforce the hypothesis that diazepam is acting through a common mechanism with calcium antagonists [75].

1.9 Pituitary gonadal axis

The paracrine and autocrine regulation within the testis as well as the endocrine interactions between the hypothalamus, the pituitary gland and the testes tightly controlled Leydig cell production of testicular androgens [76 -78]. The GnRH stimulation of gonadotropes after its binding to GnRHR, induces a biphasic increase in internal calcium with an initial spike dependent on internal calcium stores, and a sustained plateau that is dependent on increased calcium influx through calcium channels [79]. The LH is the key regulator of Leydig cell function [80,81]. Leydig cells produce testosterone necessary for both spermatogenesis and male sexual development. The endocrine control of Leydig cell steroidogenesis by LH or FSH has been exerted through their specific receptors coupled to the Ca^{2+} mediated signaling pathway [60, 61,82]. A hormonal stimulation of testicular development by FSH or LH involves a calcium influx through voltage dependent calcium channels in Sertoli cells [83,84] and Leydig cells [85]. Sertoli cells from mammalian testes are involved in the development and maintenance of spermatogenesis, support and nourishment of germ cells [86] and the synthesis and release of several proteins and a potassium rich fluid into the lumen of seminiferous tubules [87]. The gonadotropin FSH elicits a number of morphological and biochemical events in Sertoli cells by interaction with specific receptors [88]. The FSH induces changes in intracellular calcium levels [89]. Studies have suggested that FSH can influence Leydig cell function through Sertoli cells derived factors [90].

1.10 Sperm capacitation

Calcium entry through activated calcium channels causes the induction of sperm acrosome reaction . These channels are not opened in un capicitated sperm due to voltage –dependent inactivation state [91]. This inhibition can be prevented by hyperpolarization of the sperm membrane potential during the sperm capacitation process [92].

1.11 Acrosome reaction

Calcium influx is critical for the occurrence of normal acrosome reaction [93]. Acrosome reaction, the first step of fertilization, is an event allowing sperm to cross the zona pellucida and to become competent for fusion with the oocyte. The fusion of the outer acrosome membrane with the plasma membrane is dependent on the cytoplasmic calcium rise. The calcium signaling requires the successive opening and activation of different types of calcium channels such as voltage dependent calcium channels which are localized in the plasma membrane [94]. These channels represent the triggering element for the calcium signaling in sperm cells (as a calcium signaling starter) [95].

1.12 Progressive sperm motility

The new spermatozoa formed by the testes are incapable of progressive motility and consequently are unable to fertilize an egg. They gradually gain progressive motility during transit through the epididymis. Calcium is vital for their activation as sperms must swim long distances in the female reproductive tract to reach the site of fertilization [96].

1.13 Hyperactivated sperm motility

Sperms must remain in a hyperactivated state at the time and site of fertilization in order to penetrate through the gelatinous zona pellucida layer of the oocyte. Several studies indicated that calcium not only plays a role in motility but it is also an important factor in the initiation and maintenance of sperms hyperactivation [97,98].

1.14 Testicular steroidogenesis

Testosterone is synthesized in the Leydig cells of the interstitial compartment of the testes, by an enzymatic sequence of steps, from cholesterol [99]. The first and the rate- limiting step in gonadal and adrenal steroidogenesis is the transfer of the steroidogenic substrate cholesterol from the outer membrane to the inner membrane mediated by the cholesterol-transport protein, steroidogenic acute regulatory protein (StAR) [100].

1.15 Steroidogenic acute regulatory protein (StAR)

Cholesterol must transverse the aqueous space between the cholesterol – rich outer mitochondrial membrane and cholesterol poor inner mitochondrial membrane to reach the p450 side chain cleavage enzyme (CYP11A) localized within mitochondrial inner membrane in order to be converted into pregnenolone; the rate limiting step in steroid hormone synthesis. Steroid hormone biosynthesis is acutely regulated by controlling the delivery of the substrate cholesterol to P450 enzyme [101].

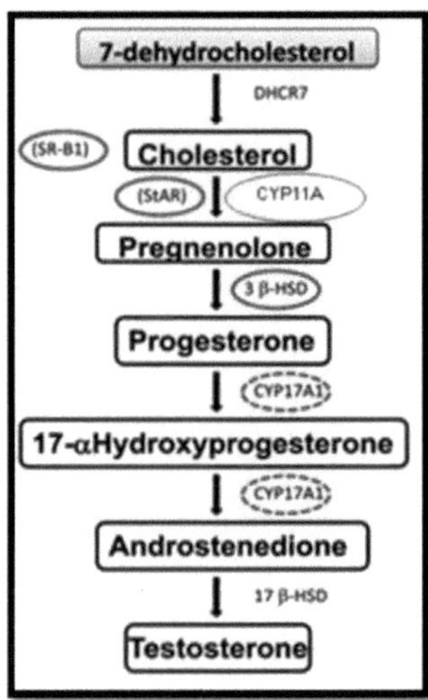

Figure (1-5) Steroid biosynthesis pathway of the testes [102]

Orme- Johnson *et al.* (1989) identified a group of mitochondrial 30 KDa phosphoproteins named the steroidogenic acute regulatory protein (StAR) that appeared in adrenal cells stimulated with ACTH and in the gonadal cells stimulated with LH [103] .These 30 KDa proteins were shown to be derived from a 37 KDa precursor synthesized in the cytoplasm and then imported into mitochondria and processed to the (StAR) proteins. The preprotein has a very short half -life (minutes) but the mature form is longer- lived (hours) [104]. In the steroidogenic cells; cholesterol serves as the substrate for the synthesis of all steroid hormones. Steroid hormones are synthesized mainly in the adrenal glands, the ovary and the testes in response to steroidogenic stimuli [105].

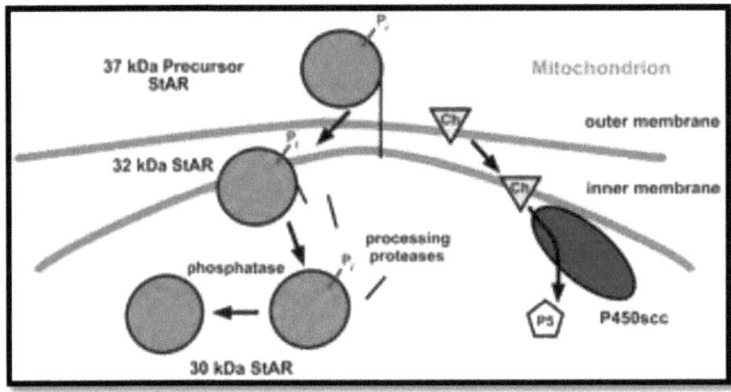

Figure (1-6) mechanism of StAR action [106]

Circulating lipoproteins are the major source of cholesterol used for steroidogenesis. Low-density lipoproteins (LDLs) are a primary reservoir of steroidogenic cholesterol, although other lipoproteins included very low density lipoproteins (VLDLs) and high density lipoproteins (HDLs) also contributing to the steroidogenic pool [107].

The peripheral-type benzodiazepine receptor or recognition site (PBR) is a widely distributed transmembrane protein that is located mainly in the outer mitochondrial membrane. The PBR binds to high-affinity drug ligands and cholesterol. Many functions are associated directly or indirectly with the PBR, including the regulation of cholesterol transport and the synthesis of steroid hormones. Translocator protein (18kDa) is proposed as a new name, regardless of the subcellular localization of the protein [108].

Current studies stated that both the steroidogenic acute regulatory protein (StAR) and the translocator protein (TSPO) have been implicated to have a concerted and indispensable effort in this cholesterol transport [109].

1.16 The StAR gene:

Steroid hormone biosynthesis is acutely regulated by pituitary trophic hormones and other steroidogenic stimuli. This regulation requires the synthesis of a protein whose function is to translocate cholesterol from the outer to the inner mitochondrial membrane in steroidogenic cells, the rate-limiting step in steroid hormone formation. The steroidogenic acute regulatory (StAR) protein is an indispensable component in this process and is the best candidate to fill the role of the putative regulator. StAR is expressed in steroidogenic tissues in response to agents that stimulate steroid production, and mutations in the StAR gene result in the disease congenital lipoid adrenal hyperplasia, in which steroid hormone biosynthesis is severely compromised. The StAR null mouse has a phenotype that is essentially identical to the human disease. The positive and negative expression of StAR is sensitive to agents that increase and inhibit steroid biosynthesis respectively. The mechanism by which StAR mediates cholesterol transfer in the mitochondria has not been fully characterized. However, the tertiary structure of the START domain of a StAR homolog has been solved, and identification of a cholesterol-binding hydrophobic tunnel within this domain raises the possibility that StAR acts as a cholesterol-shuttling protein [110].

1.17 Aim of the study

The present study was designed to evaluate the effect of diazepam treatment on the fertility status of male rats through its effects on steroidogenesis and spermatogenesis processes.

Chapter two

Materials and Methods

2.1 Drugs

The drugs used in this study are listed in table (2-1) with their production companies:

Table (2-1) List of the drugs used with their companies.

Drug	Producer
Diazepam (5mg) tablets	SDI (Iraq)
Sulfasalazine (500mg) tablets	Pharmacia (Switzerland)

2.2 Chemicals and kits

The chemicals used in this study were of the highest available purity, the specific chemicals used with their suppliers are listed in table (2-2) :

Table (2-2) List of chemicals with their suppliers

Chemicals	Supplier
Agarose powder	Biobasic (Canada)
Canada balsam natural	Win lab limited (U.K)
Diethyl ether solution	May and Baker (England)
Eosin 0.67%, nigrosin 10% stain	Merck chemical (Germany)
Ethanol (95%)	Merck (Germany)

Ethidinium bromide	Biobasic (Canada)
Formaldehyde solution (37-41)%	Merck (Germany)
Hematoxyline stain	BDH (Germany)
Loading dye (Bromophenol blue)	Geneaid (Taiwan)
Paraffin wax	Tradexpro (China)
Primers	Bioneer (Korea)
Tris-borate EDTA buffer	Biobasic (Canada)
Xylene	Merck chemical (Germany)

Kits used in this study are listed in table (2-3):

Table (2-3) List of kits with their suppliers.

Kit	Supplier
Accupower®GreenStar ^{TM} qPCR Premix	Bioneer (Korea)
Accupower®RocketScript ^{TM} RT Premix	Bioneer (Korea)
Rat FSH (ELISA) detection set	Mybiosource(USA)
Rat LH (ELISA) detection set	Cusabio (China)
Rat Testosterone (ELISA) detection set	Cusabio (China)
Total RNA mini kit (tissue)	Geneaid (Taiwan)

2.3 Instruments and tools

The instruments and tools used in this study are listed in table (2-4), with their suppliers:

Table (2-4) List of instruments with their suppliers:

Instrument	Supplier
Animal balance	China
Beakers	Duran (Germany)
Centrifuge	Kokus autech (Japan)
Cover slips	Mececo (China)
Digital balance	Mettler Toledo (Switzerland)
Digital camera	Sony (Japan)
Electronic oven	Memmert (Germany)
Electrophoresis system	Fisher Scientific (USA)
ELISA reader	Bioteck (USA)
Exicycler™ 96 Real-Time cycler	Bioneer (korea)
Eppendorf tubes (2cc)	Eppendorf (USA)
Filter paper	Whatman no.1 (UK)
Glass cylinders	Duran (Germany)
Incubator	Memmert (Germany)
Light microscope	Olympus (Japan)
Micropipette (200-1000 µl)	Volac, UK
Minispin	Eppendorf (Germany)
Minivortex	Fisher Scientific (USA)

Nanodrop	Bioneer (Korea)
Needles for oral gavage (14 Gauge, 2.9 inches (7.6cm) length, 4.0mm tip)	Kent Scientific (USA)
Neubauer hemocytometer	China
PCR thermal cycler	Fisher Scientific (USA)
Petri dish	Falcon (USA)
Sensitive balance	Sartarious (Germany)
Slides	Mececo (China)
UV transilluminator	Velber Lourmat(EEC)

2.4 Animals

50 Sprague-Dawly male rats weighing 200-250 gm and 8 weeks old were obtained from the Animal House of the College of Pharmacy-University of Baghdad. The animals were maintained on normal conditions of temperature (18°–26°C), humidity (30%–70%). and light/dark cycles (12:12) hrs. They were fed standard rodent pellet and they have free access to water.

20 Sprague-Dawly female rats weighing 200-250 gm and 8 weeks old at the estrous cycle were obtained also from the same Animal House for the study of fertility index.

2.5 Preparation of diazepam suspension

Diazepam tablets (5mg) were powdered and mixed with 5ml of distilled water, 5% carboxymethylcellulose (CMC) was added as a suspending agent to produce a suspension for different doses [111].

2.6 Preparation of sulfasalazine suspension

Sulfasalazine tablets (500mg) were powdered and mixed with 5 ml distilled water, CMC was added also as a suspending agent [112].

2.7 The study design

50 Male Rats were used in the present study, these were divided into 5 groups:

First group (control):   10 rats were administered distilled water for 8 weeks by oral gavage.

Second group (T1) : 10 rats were used for the study of the infertility activity of diazepam in which (2mg/kg B.W./day) of diazepam was given for 8 weeks by oral gavage.

Third group (T2): 10 rats were used for the study of the infertility activity of diazepam in rat model. In this group (5mg/kg B.W./day) dose of diazepam were used for 8 weeks by oral gavage.

Fourth group (T3): 10 rats were used for the study of the infertility activity of (10mg/kg B.W./day) diazepam was used for 8 weeks by oral gavage.

Fifth group (T4): 10 rats were given a dose of (500mg/kg B.W./day) of sulfasalazine for 8 weeks by oral gavage as a positive control (in this group, sulfasalazine represents standard infertility agent [113].

At the end of the treatment; two male animals from each group were mated with four females in a ratio of (1 male: 2 females) separately in isolated cages for performing the fertility index test.

Also, three male animals were taken from each group for the quantitative reverse transcriptase PCR studies.

Blood was withdrawn by cardiac puncture and was placed in a plain test tubes and left for 15 minutes then centrifuged at 3000 rpm for 15 minutes.

2.8 Determination of testes, epididymis, seminal vesicle and prostate weight to body weight ratio

After the end of the experiment period (8 weeks), the animals were weighted, anesthetized by diethyl ether. The animals were killed and testes, epididymis, seminal vesicle and prostate were obtained and weighted by sensitive balance after being cleaned from the accessory connective and adipose tissues and washed with normal saline.

The organ weight to body weight ratio was calculated according to the following equation: the organ weight to body weight ratio= weight of organ (gm)/ weight of animal (gm) ×100.

2.9 Epididymal tail suspension preparation

At the end of treatment; for each animal, the cauda epididymis was quickly removed within 5 seconds into a petridish that contains 10 ml of warm normal saline at 37°C and   it was cut longitudinally with a pair of fine pointed scissors and compressed with forceps. The sperms were released by mincing the cauda epididymis into pieces (at least 200 cuts) to perform the following microscopical examination on sperm characters [114].

2.9.1 Determination of sperm concentration

Sperm concentration was determined using the haemocytometer under light microscope (X20) objective. A cover slip was placed on the haemocytometer before a drop of the epididymal sperm solution was loaded under the cover slip[114]. Sperm count was done by counting 5 RBC small squares as shown in the following figure:

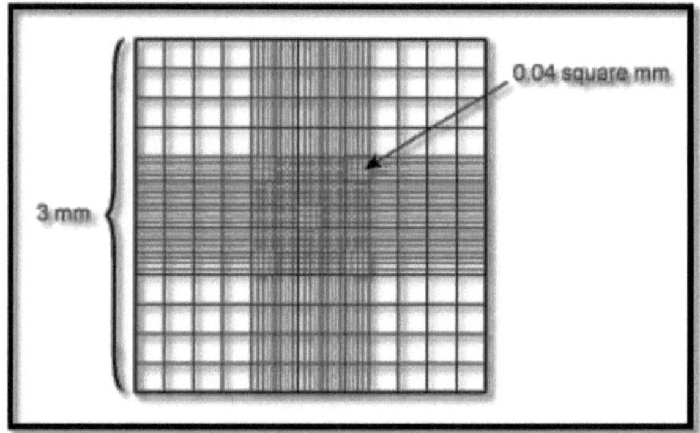

Figure (2-1) The haemocytometer under light microscope[115] .

Sperm concentration was determined using the following formula:

Sperm concentration = total no. of sperms in 5 squares ×50,000×100 (cells/ml) [114].

2.9.2 Determination of sperm motility

Sperm motility was assessed by placing a drop of the sperm suspension within 2-3 minutes over a warm clean dry slide at 37°C and covered with a cover slip and then the slide was placed under light microscope at (40X) objective. The data were tabulated in the form of percentage using the formula:

Percentage of motile sperms =no. of motile sperms ×100% / total no. of sperms (motile and immotile).

A more specified measure is motility grade, where the motility of sperm is divided into four different grades:

- **Grade a**: Sperm with progressive motility. These are the strongest and swim fast in a straight line.
- **Grade b**: (non-linear motility): These also move forward but tend to travel in a curved or crooked motion.
- **Grade c**: These have non-progressive motility because they do not move forward despite the fact that they move their tails.
- **Grade d**: These are immotile and fail to move at all [116].

2.9.3 Determination of sperm viability

In this analysis; a drop (0.05 cc) from the sperm suspension preparation   mixed with one drop (0.05cc) of eosin and then after 30 seconds, a drop (0.05cc) of nigrosin was added and mixed. Then a smear was made. After a while, the smear was air-dried and observed under light microscope (40X) objective. The dead sperms showed a pink color head while the viable sperm showed colorless or whitish head based on the degree of membrane permeability, then the data were tabulated in the form of percentage using the following formula:

Percentage of viable sperms =no. of viable sperms×100%/ total no. of dead and viable sperms [114].

2.9.4 Determination of morphologically abnormal sperms

In this analysis; the same sperm smears made for sperm viability were observed under light microscope (40X) objective. The smears were examined for abnormal morphology of the head, neck and tail. Then data were tabulated using the following formula:

Percentage of abnormal sperms =no. of abnormal sperms×100%/ total no. of normal and abnormal sperms [117].

2.10 Determination of serum LH levels

The serum levels of LH were estimated quantitatively using a readymade kit based on enzyme linked immunoassay method.

2.10.1 Principle

This kit depends on the quantitative sandwich enzyme immunoassay principle in which LH present in the standards or samples will bind to the monoclonal antibody pre-coating the microtiter plate wells. Then a standardized preparation of horseradish peroxidase (HRP) conjugated polyclonal antibody specific for LH are added to each well to sandwich the LH immobilized on the plate. Then, the microtiter plate undergoes incubation and then the wells are thoroughly washed to remove all unbound components. Later, substrate solutions are added to each well and it will react with the enzyme (HRP)   . Only those wells that contain LH and enzyme – conjugated antibody will exhibit a change in color . The enzyme – substrate reaction is terminated by addition of sulphuric acid solution as a stop solution and the color change is measured spectrophotometrically at a wave length of 450 nm in order to quantitatively measure the amount of LH present. Values of LH were expressed as (ng/ml) [118].

2.11 Determination of serum FSH levels

The serum levels of FSH were estimated quantitatively using a readymade kit based on enzyme linked immunoassay technique.

2.11.1 Principle

This assay employs the competitive enzyme immunoassay technique. The microtiter plate provided in this kit has been pre-coated with goat anti rabbit antibody. Standards or samples are added to the appropriate microtiter plate wells with an antibody specific for FSH and Horseradish Peroxidase (HRP) conjugated FSH. The competitive inhibition reaction is launched between with HRP labeled FSH and unlabeled FSH with the antibody. A substrate solution is added to the wells and the color develops in opposite to the amount of FSH in the sample. The color development is stopped and the intensity of the color is measured at 450 nm. The values were expressed as mIU/ml [119].

2.12 Determination of serum testosterone levels

The serum levels of testosterone were estimated quantitatively using a readymade kit based on enzyme linked immunoassay technique.

2.12.1 Principle

The assay of this kit employs the competitive enzyme immunoassay technique. The microtiter plate provided in this kit has been pre-coated with goat anti rabbit antibody. Standards or samples are added to the appropriate microtiter plate wells with an antibody specific for testosterone and Horseradish Peroxidase (HRP) conjugated testosterone. The competitive inhibition reaction is launched between with HRP labeled testosterone and unlabeled testosterone with the antibody. A substrate solution is added to the wells and the color develops in opposite to the amount of testosterone in the sample. The color development is stopped and the intensity of the color is measured at 450 nm. Values were expressed as ng/ml [120] .

2.13 Effect of diazepam on the fertility index

The fertility index was studied according to the method of Ratnasooriya *et al.*(2003) [121].

At the end of the treatment (8 wks); two male animals from each group were mated with four females in a ratio of (1 male: 2 females) separately in isolated cages. Before mating females were examined for the estrous cycle. Vaginal smears were obtained daily until formation of vaginal plug, stained with hematoxyline -eosin and examined under microscope. Mating was done at the estrous stage and mating was continuous for two weeks. Vaginal plug which was observed is an indication of successful mating and then females were isolated and managed until the end of pregnancy to study the reproductive indices according to the following equations:

Fertility index= no. of pregnant animals/ no. of animals mated successfully×100.

2.14 Histological Evaluation of Tissues

After the end of treatment (8 wks); the testes and epididymis were excised and cleared off from the attached fat and connective tissues. Histological sections were prepared according to Luna (1968) for histological evaluation as follows [122]:

1- Fixation: specimens were immediately fixed in 10% formalin solution in order to preserve the tissue for specimen.

2- Washing: after fixation; the specimens were washed with distilled water several times to remove the fixative,

3- Dehydration: dehydration was achieved by passing the specimens through ascending grades of ethanol (70, 80, 90 and 100%). In each run; specimen were allowed to stand in solution for 1/2 hour in order to pull the water from specimens.

4- Clearing: clearing was achieved by passing tissue through xylene.

5- Infilteration: specimens were placed in a mixture of xylene and paraffin wax at 54-56°C and then in electric oven at 60°C for 15 min. The specimens were moved to melted paraffin for 2-3 hours, during this period the paraffin were substituted each hour with a new one.

6- Embedding: the tissue block is then placed in small container of fresh, melted paraffin and removed from oven. The paraffin will solidify, encasing the tissue block.

7- Sectioning: when the paraffin solidifies; the paraffin block containing the tissue were trimmed and sectioned with microtome. Steel blade knife were used and the sections were obtained typically 5-10 µm thick.

8- Mounting: the tissue sections were fixed to a glass slide by using Mayer's albumin.

9- Staining: the histological sections were stained according to Bancroft and Stevens (1982) method [123] and as follows:

A. The paraffin was removed from sections by using xylene, on two steps and for 10 min for each step.

B. These sections were passed through different descending concentration of ethanol and finally into distilled water.

C. The sections were stained with hematoxylin for 15 min, and then washed with tap water for 10 minutes followed by distilled water washing.

D. The sections were passed through ascending concentrations of ethanol (70, 80, 90 and 100%).

E. The slides are then placed in xylene for 2 minutes.

F. Mounting: when the slides were removed from xylene, amounting medium (Balsam) that will hardens was placed over sections and a cover glass was applied.

After that the histological sections were examined under light microscope (20X and 40X) objectives.

2.15 Determination of StAR gene expression

The following PCR studies were carried out at Bioneer company representative office at Baghdad- Al-karrada. Primers were ordered from their Bioneer Corporation at Republic of Korea.

2.15.1 Extraction of RNA from tissue

Total RNA was extracted from fresh tissue (testes) using the Geneaid total RNA mini kit which was designed specifically for purifying total RNA from a variety of fresh and paraffin – embedded tissues. Tissue samples were efficiently homogenized in a microcentrifuge tube using the provided micropestle. Detergents and chaotropic salt are used to lyse cells and inactivate RNase and optional DNase treatments can be followed to remove unwanted DNA residue. RNA in the chaotropic salt is bound by the glass fiber matrix of the spin column. Once any containments have been removed, using the washing buffer (containing ethanol), the purified total RNA is eluted by RNase-free water, and is ready for use in RT-PCR [124].

2.15.2 Determination of RNA yield and purity

The most common and easiest technique to determine RNA yield and purity is absorbance using nanodrop instruments which are highly sensitive and directly provides the concentration of RNA in ng/ml. the measurement depended on the ratios of absorbance at 260 and 280 nm, i.e A260/A 280 ratio [125].

2.15.3 Conversion of RNA into cDNA using RT-PCR

The RNA extracted previously from tissues is converted into cDNA using AccuPower® Rocket Script ™ RT premix kit from Bioneer. AccuPower® Rocket Script ™ RT premix is a ready to use lyophilized master mix containing all components for first strand cDNA synthesis from a purified total RNA template. Simply by the addition of a template, primer and DEPC water to begin the reaction.

This kit contains a reverse transcriptase enzyme that has been engineered to provide increased thermal stability in order to synthesize full length first strand cDNA more efficiently, it is used to synthesize cDNA at a temperature range of 42-70°C providing increased specificity, higher yield of cDNA and more full length product [126]. The reaction is performed under the following conditions (Table 2-5):

Table (2-5) Conditions for conversion of RNA into cDNA.

Step	Temperature	Time
cDNA synthesis	42-70°C	1 hr
Heat inactivation	95 °C	5 min

The cDNA formed previously was checked using agarose gel electrophoresis. The agarose gel electrophoresis was done according to Harisha method [127]. Preparation of the agarose gel was according to Lee method [128] and the ethidium bromide staining was done according to Robinson and Lafleche method [129]. Agarose gel was visualized in a UV transilluminator and photos were captured.

2.15.4 Real time PCR (qPCR)

The cDNA was amplified using Accupower ® Green Star™ qPCR premix kit from Bioneer. Accupower®Green Star™ qPCR premix is a ready to use reagent containing all components for real- time PCR reaction just by the addition of a specific primer and target gene into tubes provides results with high sensitivity and specificity. There are three major steps at different temperatures in a PCR which are repeated for 30 or 45 cycles. Double stranded target DNA is heat denaturated (denaturation step), the two primers complementary to the target segment are annealed at low temperature (annealing step), and the annealed primers are then extended at an intermediate temperature (extension step) with a DNA polymerase. As the target copy number doubles each cycle, PCR can thereby amplify DNA fragments up to 10^8 –fold in a short period . The PCR products are detected with SYBR Green dye. SYBR Green fluorescence is enormously increased upon binding to double-stranded DNA. During the extension phase, more and more SYBR Green will bind to the PCR product resulting in an increased fluorescence. Consequently, during each subsequent PCR cycle, more fluorescence will be detected [130] . The PCR setting is shown in table (2-6).

Table (2-6) Conditions for real-time PCR

Step	Condition		Cycle
Pre-denaturation	95 °C	1min	1
Denaturation	95 °C	5 sec	40
Annealing/Extension	55°C	40 sec	
Detection(Scan)			
Melting	55°C	1 sec	1

The oligonucleotide primer sequence used for PCR amplification of StAR gene (Genebank:Access no.BC060970) is shown in table (2-7).

Table (2-7) Primer sequence for the StAR gene.

Primer	Sequences
Forward primer	LP5´-GAC CTT GAA AGG CTC AGG AAG AAC-3´
Reverse primer	RP5´-TAG CTG AAG ATG GAC AGA CTT GCC-3´

The oligonucleotide primer sequence used for PCR amplification of ß-actin gene (Genebank:Access no.NM007393) is shown in table (2-8):

Table (2-8) Primer sequence for the ß-actin gene.

Primer	Sequences
Forward primer	LP5´- ATG CCC ACT GCC GCA TCC TCT TCC -3´
Reverse primer	RP5´- CAC GAT GGA GGG GCC GGA CTC ATC-3´

The data results of qRT –PCR for the target (StAR) and housekeeping gene (ß-actin) were analyzed by the relative quantification gene expression levels (fold change) Livak method that described by [131]. In which the following formula was applicated:

Relative expression ratio= $2^{-\triangle\triangle Ct}$ and;

$\triangle\triangle$ Ct= (Ct StAR - Ct ß-actin) treatment – (Ct StAR - Ct ß-actin) control.

Ct: threshold cycle numbers

2.16 Statistical analysis

Analysis of data was carried out using the available statistical package of SPSS-21 (Statistical Packages for Social Sciences version - 21). Student t-test was used for testing the significance of difference between two groups and ANOVA for more than 2 groups. The significance of difference among different percentages (qualitative data) was tested using Chi-square test. Statistical significance was considered whenever the (p value) was equal to or less than 0.05 [132].

Chapter three

Results

3.1 Testes weight to body weight ratio

Table (3-1) showed that administration of diazepam for 8 weeks caused a highly significant decrease ($p<0.001$) in the mean testes weight to the body weight ratio of rats in the three treated groups T1 (2mg/kg), T2 (5mg/kg) and T3 (10mg/kg); (0.488 ± 0.005, 0.441 ± 0.004 and 0.389 ± 0.007) respectively, as compared with (0.526 ± 0.005) in the control group.

Also, this ratio was highly significantly ($p<0.001$) decreased in both T2 (5mg/kg); (0.441 ± 0.004) and T3 (10mg/kg) ;(0.389 ± 0.007) groups compared to T1 (2mg/kg); (0.488 ± 0.005) group. And also highly significantly ($p<0.001$) decreased in T3 (10mg/kg) ;(0.389 ± 0.007) group compared to T1 (2mg/kg); (0.488 ± 0.005) group.

The sulfasalazine group (0.358 ± 0.007) was highly significantly ($p<0.001$) reduced compared to the control, T1 (2mg/kg), T2 (5mg/kg) and T3 (10mg/kg) groups; the results were (0.526 ± 0.005, 0.488 ± 0.005, 0.441 ± 0.004 and 0.389 ± 0.007) respectively.

3.2 Epididymis weight to body weight ratio:

The present study showed that the mean epididymis weight to the body weight ratio of rats in the T1 (2mg/kg), T2 (5mg/kg), T3 (10 mg/kg) and the sulfasalazine groups was highly significantly declined compared to the control group.

Table (3-1) showed that the mean epididymis weight to the body weight ratio of rats in the T1 (2mg/kg); (0.191 ± 0.003) group was significantly ($p<0.05$) reduced as compared with the control group

(0.202±0.004), while that ratio was highly significantly (p<0.001) decreased in the T2 (5mg/kg); (0.161±0.002) and T3 (10 mg/kg) ;(0.134±0.002) groups when compared with the control (0.202±0.004) group. The ratio was highly significantly (p<0.001) decreased in both T2 (5mg/kg); (0.161±0.002) and T3 (10mg/kg); (0.134±0.002) group when compared to T1 (2mg/kg); (0.191± 0.003) group, and in T3 (10mg/kg); (0.134±0.002) group when compared to T1 (2mg/kg); (0.191± 0.003) group.

On the other hand; the sulfasalazine (0.119±0.002) group showed a highly significant (p<0.001) decrease in the epididymis to body weight ratio when compared to control, T1 (2mg/kg) and T2 (5mg/kg)groups; the results were (0.202±0.004; 0.191± 0.003 and 0.161±0.002) respectively, and a significant (p<0.05) decrease when compared to T3 10mg/kg); (0.134±0.002) group.

3.3 Seminal vesicles weight to body weight ratio:

Table (3-1) showed also the effect of diazepam on the seminal vesicles weight to body weight ratio, it showed a highly significant (p<0.001) decrease in the T1 (2mg/kg), T2 (5mg/kg) and T3 (10 mg/kg) groups as well as in the sulfasalazine group when compared to the control group. It showed a significant (p<0.05) decrease in the T1 (2mg/kg); (0.185±0.004) group when compared to the control (0.199±0.003) group. While, the T2 (5mg/kg); (0.155±0.002) group and the T3 (10mg/kg) ;(0.143±0.002) group were highly significantly (p<0.001) decreased when compared to the control (0.199±0.003) group. Also, this ratio was reduced highly significantly (p<0.001) in both the T2 (5mg/kg) ;(0.155±0.002) and T3 (10 mg/kg); (0.143±0.002) groups when compared to the T1 (2mg/kg); (0.185±0.004) group. And significantly (p<0.05) decreased in the T3 (10mg/kg); (0.143±0.002) group when compared to the T2 (5mg/kg); (0.155±0.002) group.

The sulfasalazine group (0.125±0.003) showed a highly significant (p<0.001) decline in this ratio when compared to the control, T1 (2mg/kg), T2 (5mg/kg) and T3 (10 mg/kg); the results were (0.199±0.003, 0.185±0.004, 0.155±0.002 and 0.143±0.002) respectively.

3.4 Prostate gland weight to body weight ratio:

These results showed also that the prostate gland weight to body weight ratio was highly significantly (p<0.001) decreased in the T1 (2mg/kg), T2 (5mg/kg), T3 (10 mg/kg) and the sulfasalazine groups when compared to the control group as shown in table (3-1) which showed that the effect of diazepam on the prostate weight to body weight ratio caused a significant (p<0.05) decrease in the T1 (2mg/kg) ;(0.170±0.001) group compared to the control (0.188±0.002) group, and a highly significant (p<0.001) decrease in the T2 (5mg/kg) ;(0.154±0.002) and T3 (10mg/kg) ;(0.134±0.003) groups when compared to the control (0.188±0.002) group .Also, the ratio in the T2 (5mg/kg); (0.154±0.002) group was significantly (p<0.05) reduced compared to the T1 (2mg/kg) ;(0.170±0.001) group and the T3 (10mg/kg) ;(0.134±0.003) group showed a highly significant (p<0.001) decrease in the prostate to body weight ratio compared to both T1 (2mg/kg) ;(0.170±0.001) and T2 (5mg/kg) ;(0.154±0.002) groups . The sulfasalazine (0.118±0.005) group, on the other hand; showed a highly significant (p<0.001) decrease compared to the control, T1 (2mg/kg) and T2 (5mg/kg) groups; the results were (0.188±0.002; 0.170±0.001 and 0.154±0.002) respectively, and a significant (p<0.05) decrease compared to the T3 (10 mg/kg) ;(0.134±0.003) group.

Table (3-1) The effect of different oral doses of diazepam and sulfasalazine on the testicular, epididymis, seminal vesicle and prostate gland weight to body weight ratio in male rats.

Group	Control	T1(2mg/kg)	T2(5mg/kg)	T3(10mg/kg)	Sulfasalazine (500mg/kg)
Testes/B.W ratio	0.526±0.005	0.488±0.005 *a	0.441±0.004 *a	0.389±0.007 *a	0.358±0.007 *a
Epididymis/ B.W ratio	0.202±0.004	0.191± 0.003 b	0.161±0.002 *a	0.134±0.002 *a	0.119±0.002 *ab
Seminal vesicles/B.W ratio	0.199±0.003	0.185±0.004 b	0.155±0.002 *a	0.143±0.002 *ab	0.125±0.003 *a
Prostate gland/B.W ratio	0.188±0.002	0.170±0.001 b	0.154±0.002 *ab	0.134±0.003 *a	0.118±0.005 *ab

Data are expressed as mean (±SE); n=10 rats/group. Values with different superscripts are significantly different.

3.5 Sperm concentration:

The data referring to sperm concentration in epididymal suspension of control and treated groups are shown in table (3-2).

Table (3-2): Effect of different oral doses of diazepam and sulfasalazine on the sperm concentration, motility, viability and morphology abnormalities

Group	Controls	T1(2mg/kg)	T2(5mg/kg)	T3(10mg/kg)	Sulfasalazine (500mg/kg)
Sperm conc. (million/ml)	644.5±16.2	529.9±6.56 *a	400.2±8.49 *a	292.4±9.30 *a	211±9.19 *a
Motility (%)	91.7±0.86	86.5±1.79 b	77.9± 1.83 *a	64.7± 1.85 *a	58± 1.38 *ab
Viability (%)	84.9± 1.33	81.1± 1.5	70.8± 1.65 *a	67.7± 1.01 *a	65.8± 1.16 *ab
Morphological abnormalities (%)	5.13±0.363	9.88±0.436 *a	28.24±0.923 *a	30.74±1.42 *ab	31.62±0.648 *ab

Data are expressed as mean (±SE); n=10 rats/group. Values with different superscripts are significantly different.

The present study showed that the sperm concentration was highly significantly (p< 0.001) reduced in the T1 (2mg/kg), T2 (5mg/kg) and T3 (10mg/kg) groups, the results were (529.9± 6.56 million/ ml; 400.2± 8.49 million/ ml and 292.4±9.30 million/ ml) respectively as compared to the control (644.5±16.29 million/ml) group. And was also highly significantly (p< 0.001) declined in the T2 (5mg/kg); (400.2±8.49 million/ml) and T3 (10mg/kg) ;(292.4±9.30million/ml) groups as compared to the T1 (2mg/ml) ;(529.9±6.56 million/ml) group. And in the T3 (10 mg/kg); (292.4±9.30million/ml) as compared to the T2 (5mg/kg); (400.2±8.49 million/ml) group. While the sperm concentration in the sulfasalazine group ;(211±9.19 million/ml) was also highly significantly (p< 0.001) decreased as compared to the control, T1 (2mg/kg), T2 (5mg/kg) and T3 (10 mg/kg) groups; (644.5±16.29million/ml; 529.9±6.56million/ml; 400.2±8.49million/ml and 292.4±9.30million/ml) respectively.

3.6 Sperm motility:

Table (3-2) showed that after 8 weeks of diazepam treatment, the sperm motility in the T1 (2mg/kg), T2 (5mg/kg), T3 (10 mg/kg) and in the sulfasalazine group were highly significantly decreased compared to the control group. The results showed a significant decrease (p< 0.05) in sperm motility in the T1 (2mg/kg); (86.5±1.79%) group as compared to the control (91.7±0.86%) group while the T2 (5mg/kg); (77.9± 1.83%) and the T3 (10mg/kg); (64.7± 1.85%) groups showed a highly significant (p< 0.001) decrease as compared to the control (91.7±0.86%) group. Also, the T2 (5mg/kg); (77.9± 1.83%) and the T3 (10mg/kg); (64.7± 1.85%) groups showed a highly significant (p< 0.001) decrease as compared to the T1 (2mg/kg) ;(86.5±1.79%) group. And the T3 (10mg/kg); (64.7± 1.85%) group was also highly significantly (p< 0.001) decreased compared to the T2 (5mg/kg); (77.9± 1.83%) group. On the other hand, the sulfasalazine ;(58± 1.38%) group was highly significantly (p< 0.001) decreased compared to the control (91.7±0.86%) , T1 (2mg/kg); (86.5±1.79%) and T2 (5mg/kg); (77.9± 1.83%) groups and significantly (p< 0.05) decreased compared to the T3 (10 mg/kg); (64.7± 1.85%) group.

3.7 Sperm viability:

The effect of diazepam on the percentage of dead sperms is shown in table (3-2). There was no significant difference in the viability percentage between the control (84.9± 1.33%) group and T1 (2mg/kg); (81.1± 1.5%) group. But, there was a highly significant (p< 0.001) decrease in both T2 (5mg/kg); (70.8± 1.65%) and T3 (10 mg/kg); (67.7± 1.01%) groups compared to the control (84.9± 1.33%) and T1 (2mg/kg); (81.1± 1.5%) groups. Also there was no significant difference between T3 (10 mg/kg); (67.7± 1.01%) and T2 (5mg/kg); (70.8± 1.65%) groups. The sulfasalazine (65.8± 1.16%) group showed a highly significant (p< 0.001) decrease compared to the control (84.9± 1.33%) and T1 (2mg/kg); (81.1± 1.5%) groups, a significant (p< 0.05) decrease compared to the T2(5mg/kg); (70.8± 1.65%) group and no significant decrease compared to the T3(10 mg/kg); (67.7± 1.01%) group.

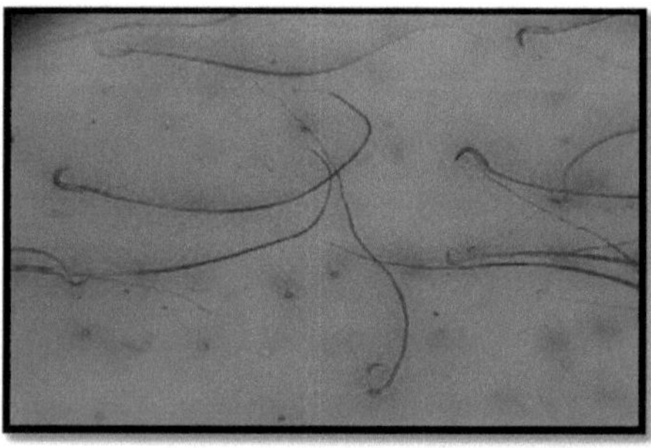

Figure (3-1) Sperm viability (X40)

3.8 Morphologically abnormal sperms:

The results of the morphologically abnormal shaped sperms are shown in table (3-2) also. After 8 weeks of the treatment; the percentage of the morphologically abnormal sperms increased highly significantly (p< 0.001) in the T1 (2mg/kg), T2 (5mg/kg) and T3 (10mg/kg) groups compared to the control group.

The present study showed that the percentage of morphologically abnormal sperms was highly significantly (p< 0.001) increased in the T1 (2mg/kg), T2 (5 mg/kg) and T3 (10 mg/kg) groups; the results were (9.88±0.436 %; 28.24±0.923% and 30.74±1.42%) respectively compared to the control (5.13±0.363%) group. And it was also highly significantly (p< 0.001) increased in both T2 (5mg/kg); (28.24±0.923%) and T3 (10 mg/kg); (30.74±1.42%) groups compared toT1(2mg/kg) ;(9.88±0.436%). Also, it was significantly (p< 0.05) increased in T3 (10 mg/kg); (30.74±1.42%) group compared to T2 (5mg/kg); (28.24±0.923%) group. In the sulfasalazine (31.62±0.648%) group the percentage of the morphologically abnormal sperms was highly significantly (p< 0.001) increased compared to the control (5.13±0.363) and T1 (2mg/kg) ;(9.88±0.436%) groups but significantly (p< 0.05) increased compared to T2 (5mg/kg); (28.24±0.923%) group. And it was not significantly different from that of the T3 (10 mg/kg); (30.74±1.42%) group.

Figure (3-2, A) showed the normal shape sperms while figures (3-2, B, C, D, E and F) showed the main abnormal shapes of sperms caused by the drug.

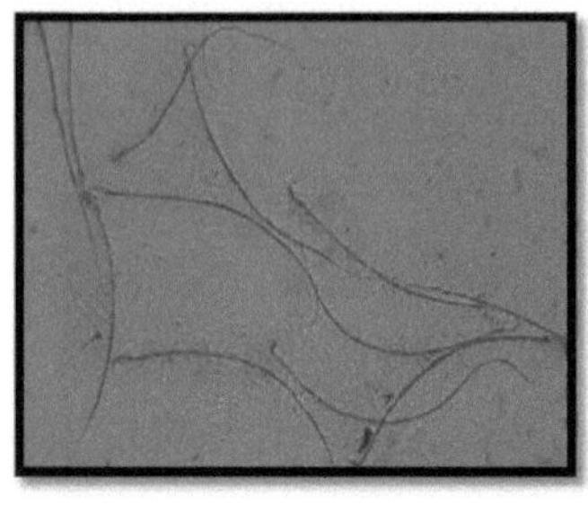

(3-2,A) Normal shape sperms (X40).

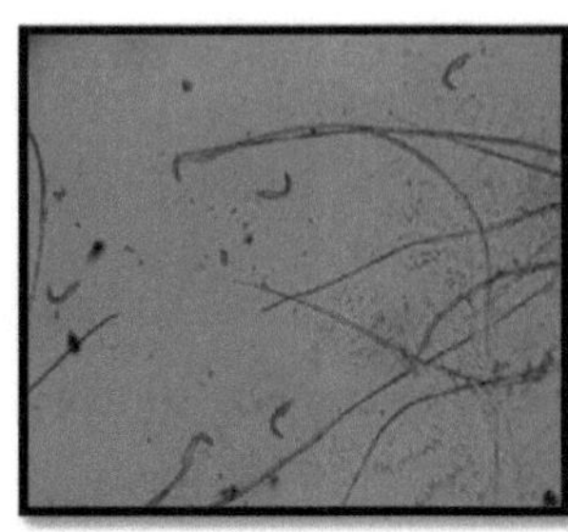

(3-2,B)Tailless sperms (X40).

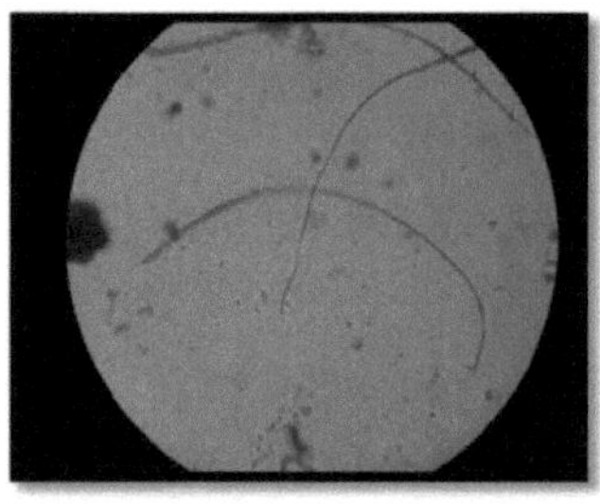

(3-2,C) Headless sperms (X40).

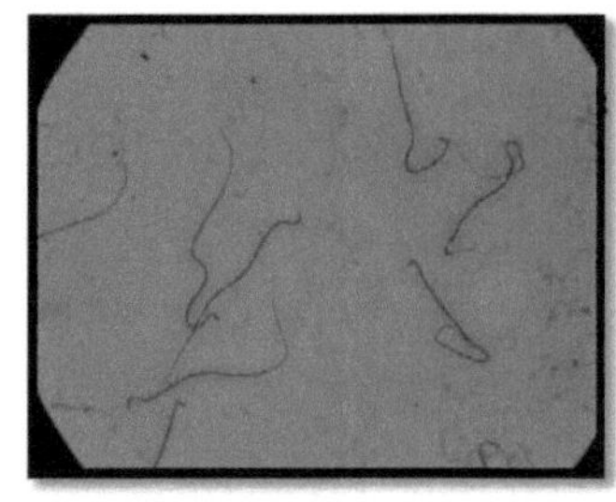

(3-2,D) Bent mid- tail sperms (X40).

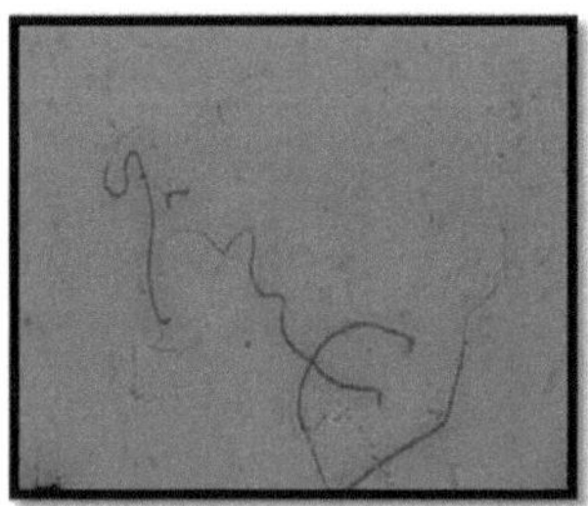

(3-2,E) Abnormal long tail sperms (X40).

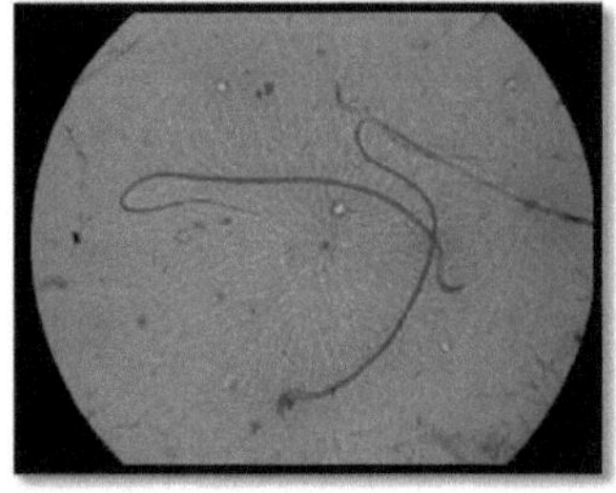

(3-2,F) Coiled tail sperms (X40).

3.9 Grades of motility:

The data referring to the effect of drug on grades of sperms motility are shown in table (3-3).

Table (3-3): Effect of different oral doses of diazepam on the grades of motility in male rats.

Group	Control	T1(2mg/kg)	T2(5mg/kg)	T3(10mg/kg)	Sulfasalazine (500mg/kg)
Progressive motility;(%) Grade a	38.2±1.61	35.3± 1.8	24.1±1.48 *a	16.1± 1.68 *ab	14.6± 1.23 *a
Circular motility (%) Grade b	40.7± 2.3	37.9± 1.87	32.2± 2.37 b	23.7± 2.05 *ab	19.9± 0.948 *a
Insitu motility (%) Grade c	12.8±3.29	13.3±2.02	21.6± 1.85 b	24.9±3.06 b	23.5±1.34 b
Immotile (%) Grade d	8.3± 0.86	13.5±1.7 b	22.1± 1.83 *a	35.3± 1.85 *a	42± 1.38 *ab

Data are expressed as mean (±SE); n=10 rats/group. Values with different superscripts are significantly different.

Table (3-3) showed that there was no significant difference in the progressive motility percentage between control (38.2±1.61%) group and T1 (2mg/kg) ;(35.3± 1.8%).While, there was a highly significant (p< 0.001) decrease in the progressive motility percentage between both T2 (5mg/kg); (24.1±1.48%) and T3 (10mg/kg); (16.1± 1.68%) compared to control group; (38.2±1.61%). Also, there was a highly significant (p< 0.001) decrease in the progressive motility percentage between both T2 (5mg/kg) ;(24.1±1.48%) and T3 (10 mg/kg); (16.1± 1.68%) compared to T1 (2mg/kg) ;(35.3± 1.8%). While the T3 (10 mg/kg); (16.1± 1.68%) group showed a significant (p< 0.05) decrease compared to T2 (5mg/kg); (24.1±1.48%) group. On the other hand, the sulfasalazine (14.6± 1.23%) group showed a highly significant (p< 0.001) decrease in the progressive motility percentage compared to control, T1 (2mg/kg) and T2 (5mg/kg); (38.2±1.61%; 35.3± 1.8% and 24.1±1.48%) respectively. And, also showed no significant decrease compared to T3 (10mg/kg); (16.1± 1.68%) group.

Considering the curve motility; there was no significant difference between control group; (40.7± 2.3%) and T1 (2mg/kg); (37.9± 1.87%), while there was a significant (p< 0.05) difference between T2 (5mg/kg); (32.2± 2.37%) and both the controls; (40.7± 2.3%) and T1 (2mg/kg); (37.9± 1.87%). The T3 (10 mg/kg); (23.7± 2.05%) group showed a highly significant (p< 0.001) decrease compared to control; (40.7± 2.3%) and T1 (2mg/kg); (37.9± 1.87%) and a significant (p< 0.05) decrease compared to T2 (5mg/kg). The sulfasalazine group (19.9± 0.948%) was highly significantly (p< 0.001) decreased compared to control , T1 (2mg/kg) and T2 (5mg/kg); (40.7± 2.3%, 37.9± 1.87% and 32.2± 2.37%) respectively. while there was no significant difference between the sulfasalazine group (19.9± 0.948%) and the T3 (10 mg/kg); (23.7± 2.05%) group.

Insitu motility; there was no significant difference between control; (12.8±3.29%) and T1 (2mg/kg); (13.3±2.02%) group but there was a significant (p< 0.05) difference between control; (12.8±3.29%) compared to T2 (5mg/kg) and T3 (10mg/kg) groups; (21.6± 1.85%) and (24.9±3.06%) respectively.

The T2 (5mg/kg); (21.6± 1.85%) and T3 (10 mg/kg); (24.9±3.06%) groups were increased significantly (p< 0.05) compared to T1 (2mg/kg); (13.3±2.02%) group. While there was no significant difference between T2 (5mg/kg); (21.6± 1.85%) and T3 (10 mg/kg); (24.9±3.06%) groups. On the other hand, the sulfasalazine ;(23.5±1.34%) group showed a significant (p< 0.05) increase compared to both the control; (12.8±3.29%) and T1 (2mg/kg); (13.3±2.02%) groups. While it shows no significant difference compared to both T2 (5mg/kg) ;(21.6± 1.85%) and T3 (10 mg/kg); (24.9±3.06%) groups

According to the percentage of immotile sperms; there was a significant (p< 0.05) increase in the percentage of immotile sperms in the T1 (2mg/kg); (13.5±1.7%) group compared to control (8.3± 0.86%) group. While both the T2 (5 mg/kg); (22.1± 1.83%) and T3 (10 mg/kg); (35.3± 1.85%) groups showed a highly significant (p< 0.001) increase compared to control (8.3± 0.86%) and also, both the T2 (5mg/kg);(22.1± 1.83%) and T3(10mg/kg); (35.3± 1.85%) groups showed a highly significant (p< 0.001) increase compared to T1 (2mg/kg); (13.5±1.7%). The T3 (10mg/kg); (35.3± 1.85%) group showed a highly significant (p< 0.001) increase compared to T2 (5 mg/kg); (22.1± 1.83%) group. Considering the sulfasalazine ;(42± 1.38%) group, there was a highly significant (p< 0.001) increase in the percentage of immotile sperms compared to controls (8.3± 0.86%) , T1 (2mglkg); (13.5±1.7%) and T2 (5mg/kg);(22.1± 1.83%) groups but a significant (p< 0.05) increase compared to T3(10mg/kg); (35.3± 1.85%) group.

3.10 Serum LH levels:

The data referring to the effect of the drug on serum LH,FSH and testosterone are shown in table (3-4):

Table (3-4): Effect of different oral doses of diazepam on the serum levels of hormones in male rats.

Group	Control	T1(2mg/kg)	T2(5mg/kg)	T3(10mg/kg)	Sulfasalazine (500mg/kg)
LH (ng/ml)	12.02±0.235	9.59± 0.193 *a	5.28±0.152 *a	2.7± 0.149 *a	2.24± 0.85 *a
FSH (mIU/ml)	20.99±0.468	18.34±0.282 *a	16.58±0.254 *a	14.27±0.324 *a	12.16±0.233 *a
Testosterone (ng/ml)	5.13±0.221	4.0±0.092 *a	3.16±0.085 *a	2.52±0.103 *ab	1.8±0.129 *a

Data are expressed as mean (±SE); n=10 rats/group. Values with different superscripts are significantly different.

The results in table (3-4) showed that serum LH levels was highly significantly (p< 0.001) reduced in the three treatment doses T1 (2mg/kg), T2 (5mg/kg), T3 (10mg/kg) and in the sulfasalazine group compared to the control group. It showed that the serum LH level was highly significantly(p< 0.001) decreased in the T1 (2mg/kg), T2 (5mg/kg) and T3 10 mg/kg) groups; the results were (9.59± 0.193ng/ml, 5.28±0.152 ng/ml and 2.7± 0.149 ng/ml) respectively; compared to the control (12.02±0.235ng/ml) group , and it was highly significantly(p< 0.001) reduced in both T2 (5mg/kg); (5.28±0.152ng/ml) and T3 (10 mg/kg); (2.24± 0.85 ng/ml) compared to the T1(2mg/kg);(9.59± 0.193ng/ml) group. And in the T3 (10 mg/kg); (2.24± 0.85 ng/ml) group compared to the T2 (5mg/kg); (5.28±0.152ng/ml) group. While the serum LH levels was highly significantly (p< 0.001) reduced in the sulfasalazine (2.24± 0.85ng/ml) group compared to the control, T1 and T2 groups; the results were (12.02±0.235ng/ml, 9.59± 0.193ng/ml and 5.28±0.152ng/ml) respectively with no significant difference compared to the T3 (10 mg/kg); (2.24± 0.85 ng/ml) group.

3.11 Serum FSH levels:

The present study showed that the serum FSH levels was highly significantly (p< 0.001) reduced in the T1 (2mg/kg), T2 (5mg/kg), T3 (10mg/kg) and in the sulfasalazine group compared to the control group. Table (3-4) showed that serum FSH levels was highly significantly (p< 0.001) reduced in the T1 (2mg/kg), T2 (5mg/kg) and T3 (10mg/kg) groups; the results were (18.34±0.282 mIU/ml, 16.58±0.254 mIU/ml and 14.27±0.324 mIU/ml) respectively; compared to the control (20.99±0.468 mIU/ml) group. And it was highly significantly (p< 0.001) reduced in both T2 (5mg/kg) ; (16.58±0.254 mIU/ml)   and T3(10 mg/kg); (14.27±0.324 mIU/ml) groups compared to T1(2mg/kg) ; (18.34±0.282 mIU/ml) group. Also, in the T3 (10 mg/kg); (14.27±0.324 mIU/ml) group compared to the T2 (5mg/kg); (16.58±0.254 mIU/ml) group .While the sulfasalazine (12.16±0.233) group showed a highly significant (p< 0.001) reduction compared to the control, T1, T2 and T3; the results were (20.99±0.468 mIU/ml, 18.34±0.282 mIU/ml, 16.58±0.254 mIU/ml and 14.27±0.324 mIU/ml groups.

3.12 Serum testosterone levels:

The present study showed that serum testosterone levels was highly significantly (p< 0.001) reduced in the T1 (2mg/kg), T2 (5mg/kg), T3 (10mg/kg) and the sulfasalazine group as compared to the control group as shown in table (3-4) which showed that the serum levels of testosterone hormone were highly significantly (p< 0.001) reduced in the T1 (2mg/kg) , T2 (5mg/kg) and T3(10 mg/kg); the results were (4.0±0.092ng/ml, 3.16±0.085ng/ml and 2.52±0.103ng/ml) respectively as compared to the control (5.13±0.221ng/ml) group. While the serum levels of testosterone in the T2 (5mg/kg);(3.16±0.085ng/ml) and T3(10mg/ml); (2.52±0.103 ng/ml) groups were highly significantly (p< 0.001) reduced as compared to the T1(2mg/kg);(4.0±0.092 ng/ml) group, but the serum levels of testosterone were significantly(p< 0.05) reduced in the T3 (10mg/ml); (2.52±0.103 ng/ml) group as compared to the T2(5mg/kg);   (3.16±0.085ng/ml)   group.   The   sulfasalazine (1.8±0.129ng/ml) group on the other hand; was highly significantly (p< 0.001) reduced compared to the control, T1, T2 and T3 groups; the results were   (5.13±0.221ng/ml,   4.0±0.092ng/ml,   3.16±0.085ng/ml   and 2.52±0.103ng/ml) respectively.

3.13 Fertility index:

The effect of the three doses of diazepam given orally to male rats mated with non treated females showed that there was significant changes (p<0.05) in the percentage of fertility index among the four groups using chi-square analysis. The results showed that the fertility index was (100%) in the control group, (50%) in T1 group, (25%) in T2 group, (25%) in T3 group and (25%) in the sulfasalazine group as shown in table (3-5).

Table (3-5): Effect of different oral doses of diazepam on the fertility index.

Group	Control	T1(2mg/kg)	T2(5mg/kg)	T3(10mg/kg)	Sulfasalazine (500mg/kg)
No. of females mated successfully	4	4	4	4	4
No. of pregnant animals	4	2	1	1	1
Fertility index (%)	100%	50% b	25% b	25% b	25% b

Data are expressed as(%). Values with different superscripts are significantly different.

These results showed that the fertility index was significantly (p<0.05) decreased in the T1 (2mg/kg), T2 (5mg/kg), T3 (10 mg/kg) and the sulfasalazine group compared to the control group; the results were (50%, 25%, 25% and 25 %) respectively compared to the control (100%) group. Also, the fertility index in the T2 (5mg/kg), T3 (10 mg/kg) and the sulfasalazine group was significantly (p<0.05) lower than T1 group; the results were (25%, 25% and 25%) respectively compared to(50%) in the T1 group (2mg/kg) .On the other hand ; there was no significant difference between T2 (5mg/kg); (25%) and T3 (10mg/kg); (25%) and the sulfasalazine group;(25%).

3.14 The histological changes in testicular and epididymal tissues:

The microscopic study of rat testes and epididymis treated with diazepam for 8 weeks revealed variable degrees of alteration according to the dose of treatment compared to the control group. Many histological changes in semniferous tubules, spermatogenesis and number of sperms in the lumen of semniferous tubules are occurred.

Figures (3-3, A and B) show sections of the control rat testis with normal structure appearance of semniferous tubules and full maturation of spermatogonia cells and sperms present inside the lumen (normal spermatogenesis).

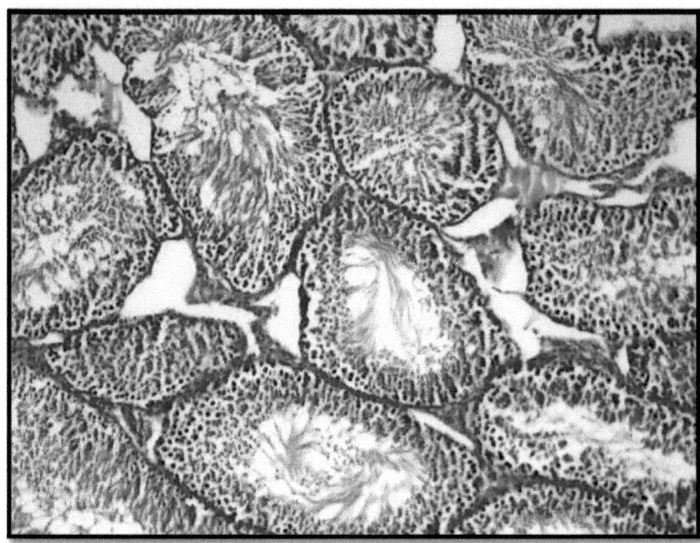

Figure (3-3, A) Cross section of normal rat´s testes (control group), (H& E×20).

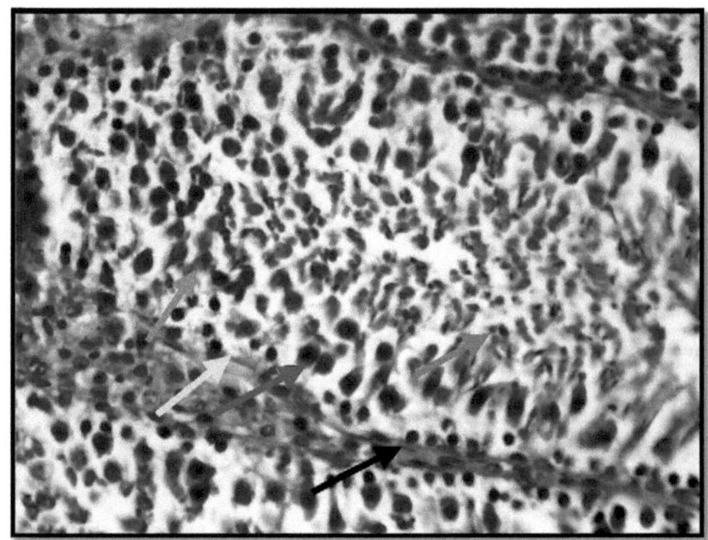

Figure (3-3, B) Cross section of normal rat´s testes (control group), black arrow shows spermatogonia, red arrow shows primary spermatocytes, blue arrow shows secondary spermatocytes, green arrow shows spermatids and yellow arrow shows sertoli cells (H& E ×40).

While figures (3-4, A and B) show sections of epididymis in the control rat. It shows normal structure of tubules lined by columnar epithelial cells with sterocilla containing a collection of sperms inside the lumen.

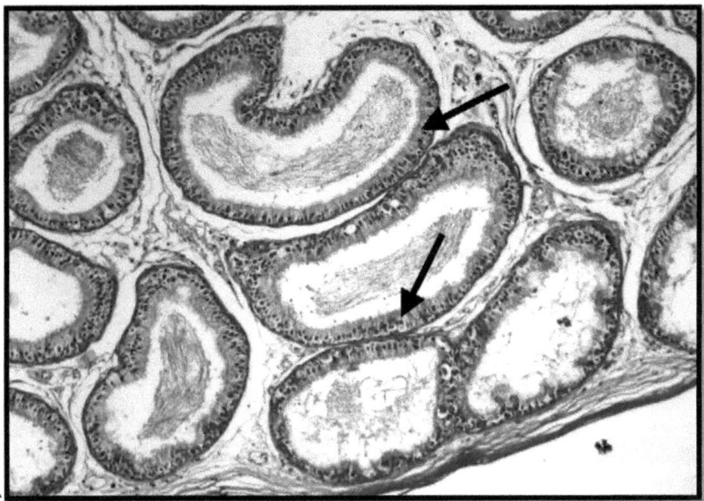

Figure (3-4, A) Cross section of normal rat′s epididymis (control group), black arrows show pseudostratified columnar epithelial cells (H&E ×20).

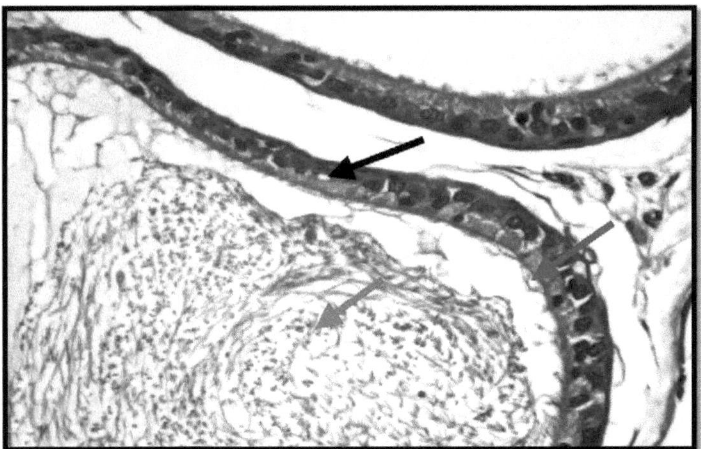

Figure (3-4, B) Cross section of normal rat′s epididymis (control group), black arrow shows pseudostratified columnar epithelium cells, red arrow shows sterocilla, green arrow shows sperms inside lumen, (H&E ×40) .

Figures (3-5, A and B) show sections of rat´s testis treated with 2mg/kg of diazepam in which certain semniferous tubules are empty from the production of sperms.

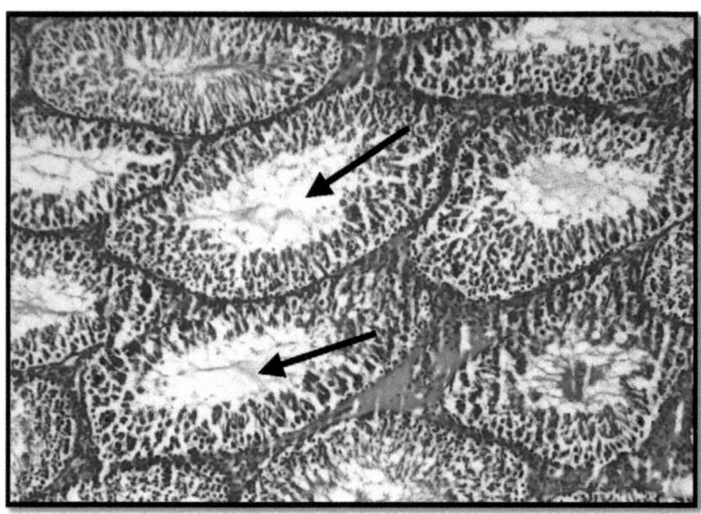

Figure (3-5, A) Cross section of rat´s testes treated with 2 mg/Kg of diazepam , black arrows showing few sperms, (H&E ×20) .

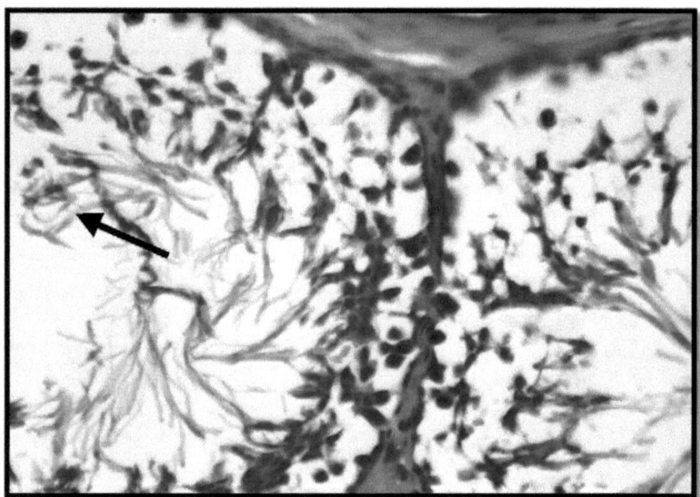

Figure (3-5, B) Cross section of rat´s testis treated with 2 mg/Kg of diazepam , black arrow shows few sperms, (H&E ×40) .

Figures (3-6,A and B) show sections of rat´s epididymis treated with 2mg/kg of diazepam in which some of the epididymal tubules showing no contents of sperms and other showing few sperm transport.

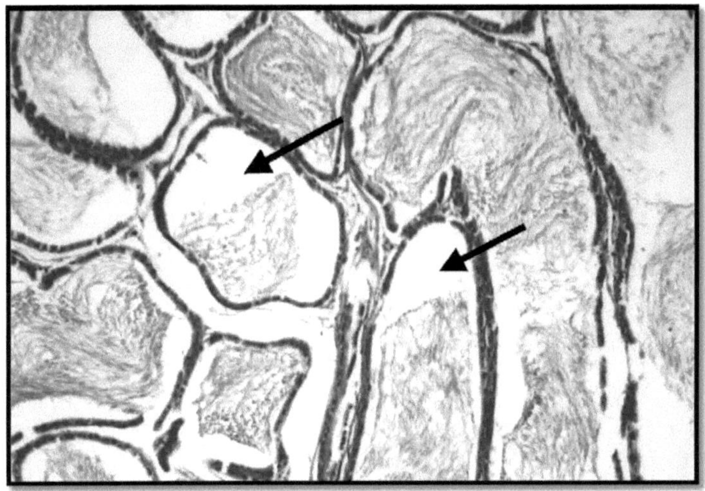

Figure (3-6, A) Cross section of rat´s epididymis treated with 2 mg/Kg of diazepam , black arrows show no sperms, (H&E ×20).

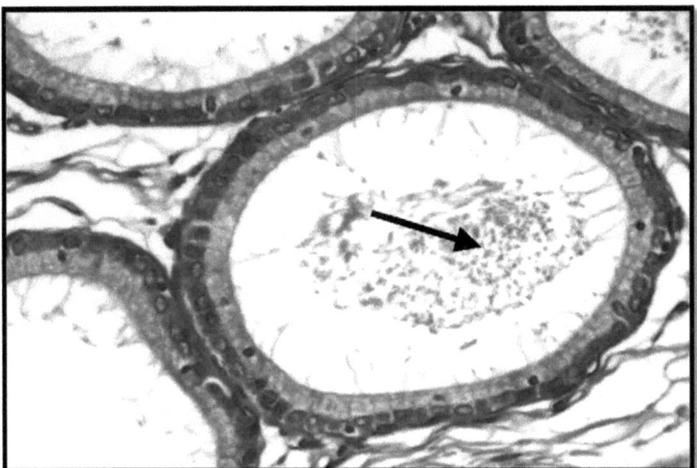

Figure (3-6, B) Cross section of rat´s epididymis treated with 2 mg/Kg of diazepam , black arrow showing few sperms (H&E ×40) .

Figures (3-7 ,A and B) show sections of rat's testis treated with 5mg/kg of diazepam in which certain tubules show damage of maturity of sperm production cells (primary spermatocytes, secondary spermatocytes and spermatids).

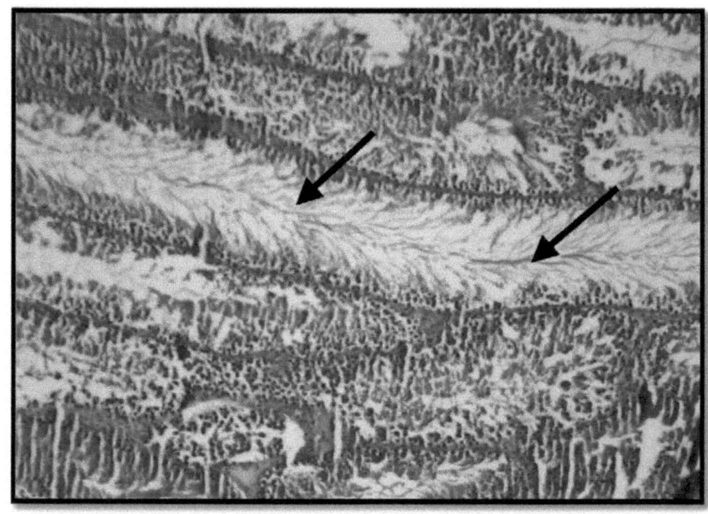

Figure (3-7, A) Longitudinal section of rat's testis treated with 5 mg/Kg of diazepam , black arrows show no sperms (H&E ×20).

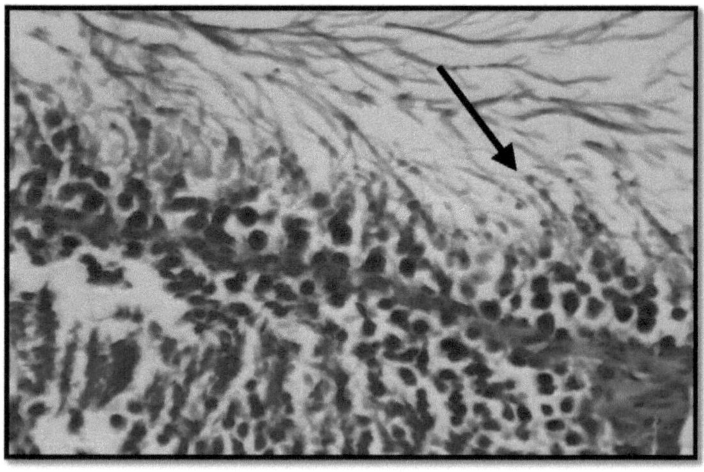

Figure (3-7, B) Cross section of rat's testis treated with 5mg/Kg of diazepam , black arrow shows few sperms (H&E ×40).

Figures (3-8, A and B) show sections of rat's epididymis treated with 5mg/kg of diazepam in which certain tubules show few or no sperms.

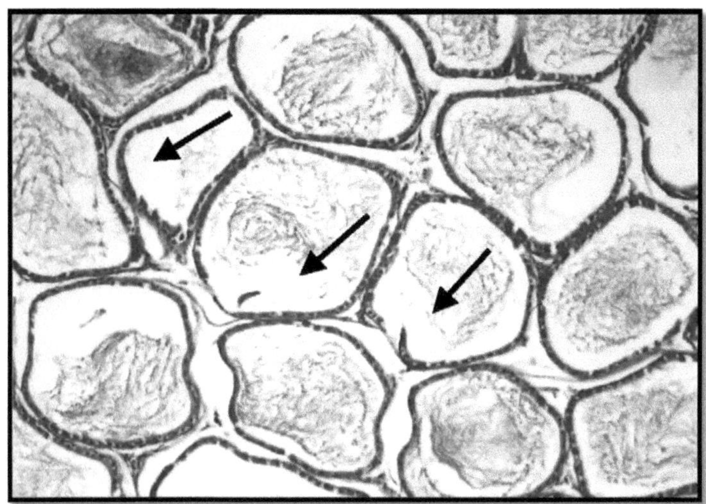

Figure (3-8, A) Cross section of rat 's epididymis treated with 5 mg/Kg of diazepam , black arrows showing few or no sperms (H&E ×20).

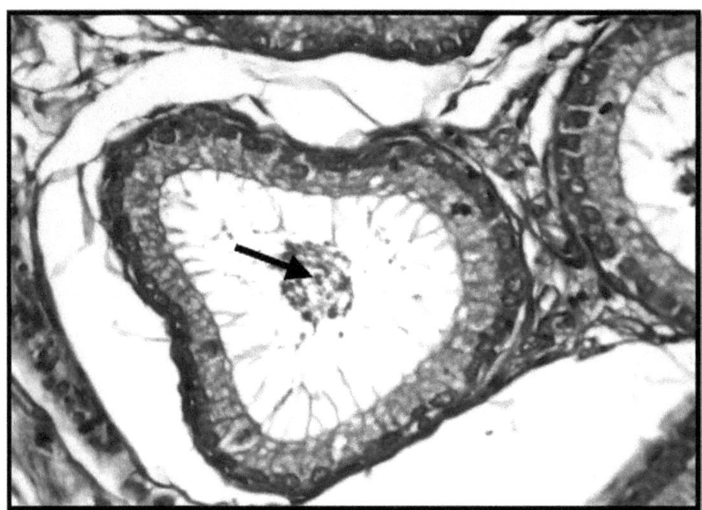

Figure (3-8, B) Cross section of rat's epididymis treated with 5 mg/Kg of diazepam , black arrows showing few sperms (H&E ×40).

Figures (3-9, A and B) show sections of rat's testis treated with 10mg/kg of diazepam in which there is some severe necrosis of products with certain necrosis of spermatogenic cells, other show no products of sperm.

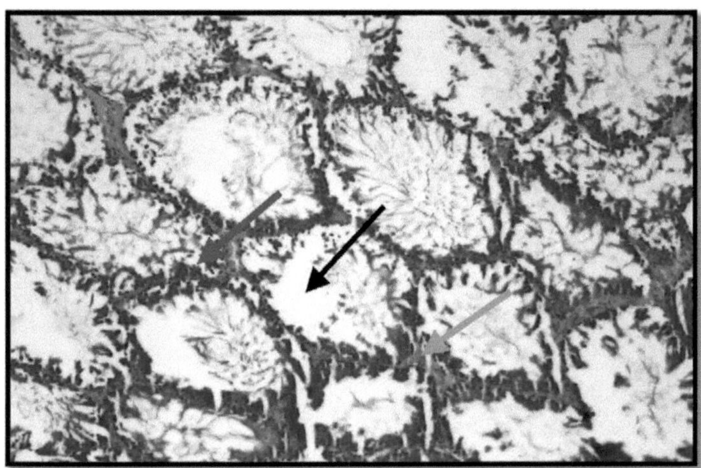

Figure (3-9, A) Cross section of rat's testis treated with 10 mg/Kg of diazepam , black arrows shows no products of sperms, green arrow shows Leydig cell atrophy, red arrow shows decreased number of sertoli cells (H&E ×20).

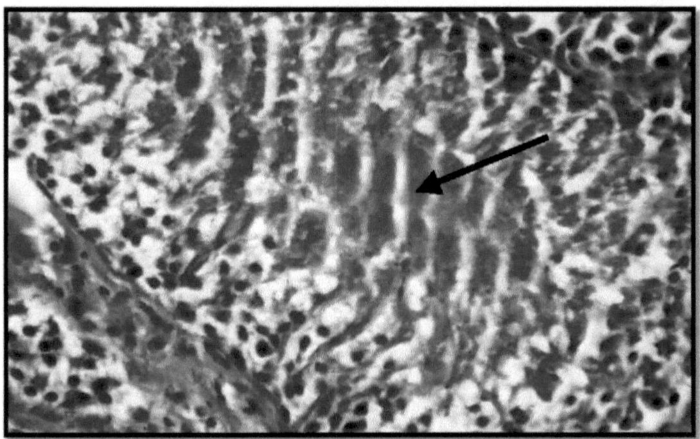

Figure (3-9, B) Cross section of rat's testis treated with 10 mg/Kg of diazepam , black arrow shows spermatogenic cell necrosis, (H&E ×40).

Figures (3-10,A and B) show sections of rat´s epididymis treated with 10mg/kg of diazepam in which some of the epididymal tubules contains few sperms inside the lumen.

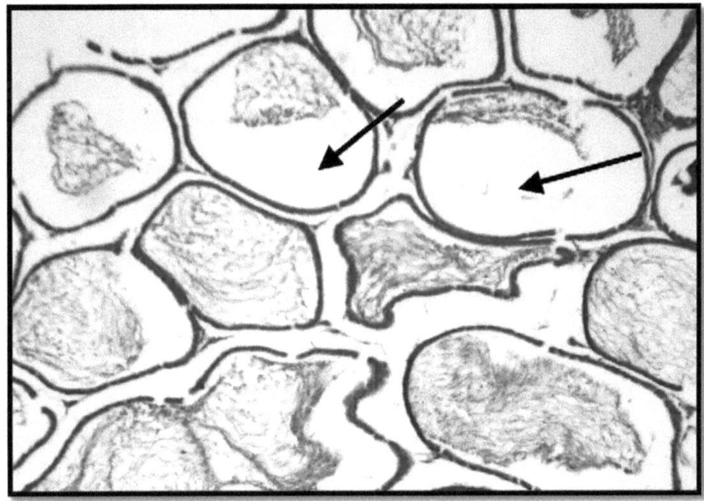

Figure (3-10, A) Cross section of rat´s epididmyis treated with 10 mg/Kg of diazepam , black arrows showing few or no sperms inside the lumen(H&E ×20).

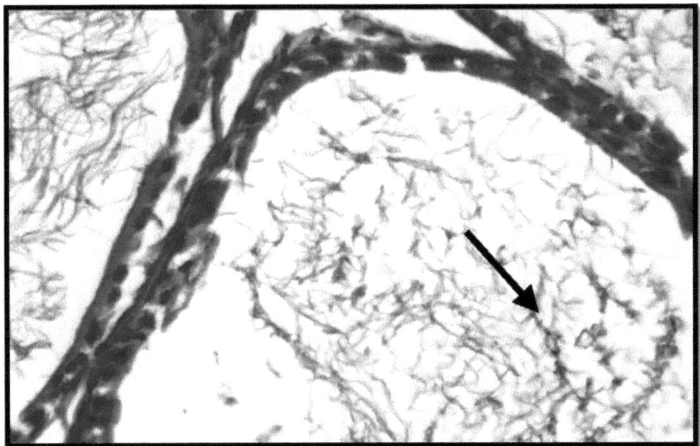

Figure (3-10, B) Cross section of rat´s epididmyis treated with 10 mg/Kg of diazepam , black arrow shows few or no sperms inside the lumen, (H&E ×40) .

Figures (3-11, A and B) show sections of rat´s testis treated with sulfasalazine showing immaturation of spermatogonia cells with few sperms inside the lumen.

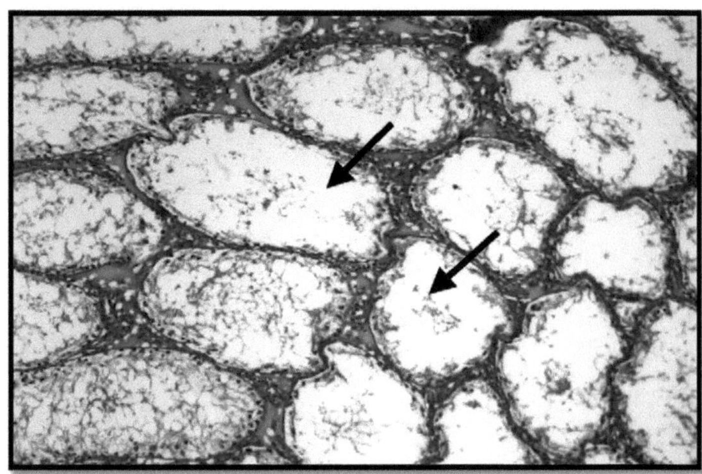

Figure (3-11, A): Cross section of rat´s testis treated with sulfasalazine, black arrows show damage of semniferous tubules & loss of spermatogenesis (H&E ×20)

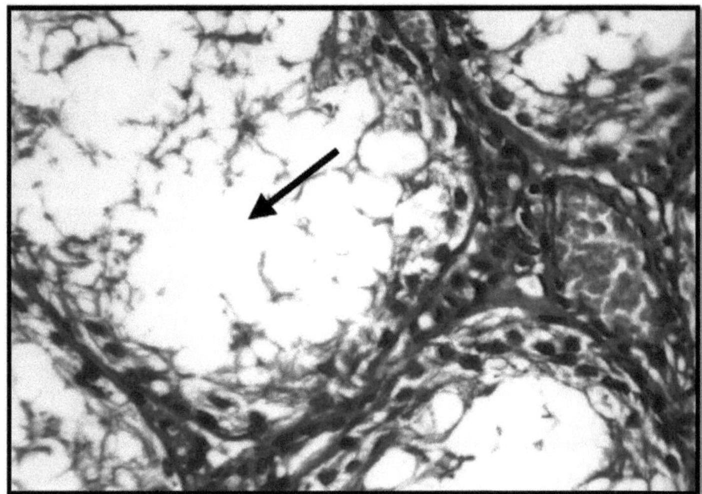

Figure (3-11, B) Cross section of rat ´s testis treated with sulfasalazine, black arrow shows few or no sperms inside lumen (H&E ×40)

Figures (3-12, A and B) show sections of rat's epididymis treated with sulfasalazine showing few collections of sperms inside the lumen.

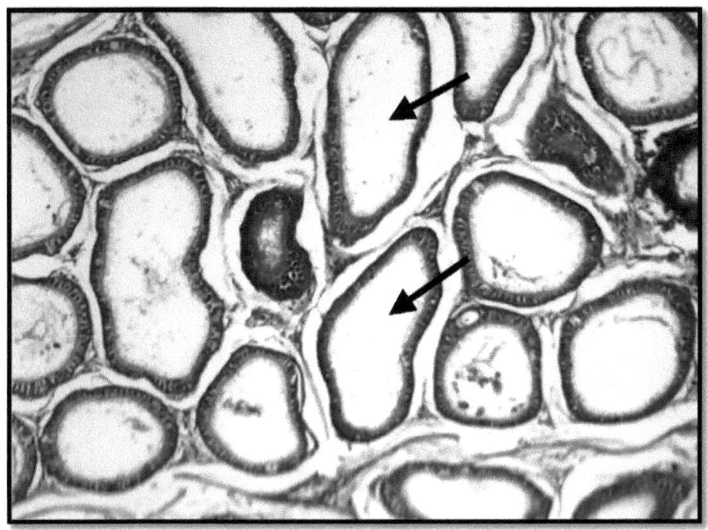

Figure (3-12, A) Cross section of rat epididymis treated with sulfasalazine, black arrows show few or no sperms inside lumen (H&E ×20)

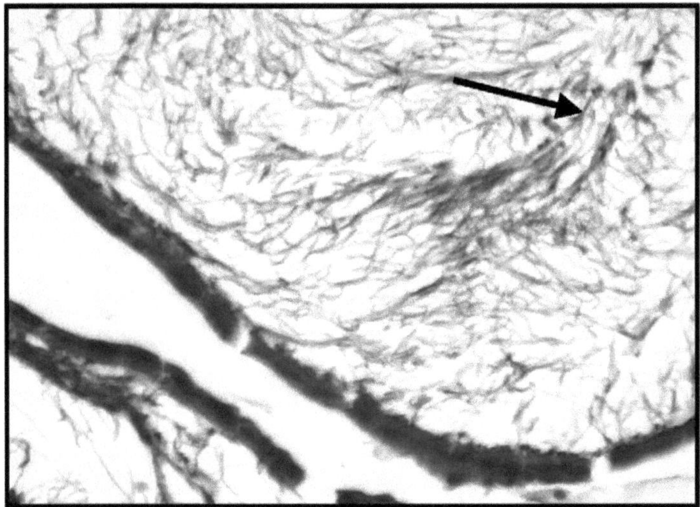

Figure (3-12, B) Cross section of rat epididymis treated with sulfasalazine Black arrow shows few sperms (H&E ×40).

3.15 Quantitative Reverse transcriptase Real – time PCR:

Quantitative Reverse transcriptase Real – time PCR (RT-q PCR) was performed for measurement of relative quantification (gene expression analysis) for StAR gene expression level normalized by housekeeping gene expression (ß-actin). Reverse transcriptase Real – time PCR quantification method was dependent on the values threshold cycle numbers (CT) of amplification plot of target gene and housekeeping gene. The results are shown in figures (3-13, A&B) for control group, figures (3-14, A&B) for T1 group ;(2mg/kg) of diazepam , figures (3-15,A &B) for T2 group; (5mg/kg) of diazepam , figures (3-16, A&B) for T3 group; (10mg/kg) of diazepam and figures (3-17, A&B) for sulfasalazine group.

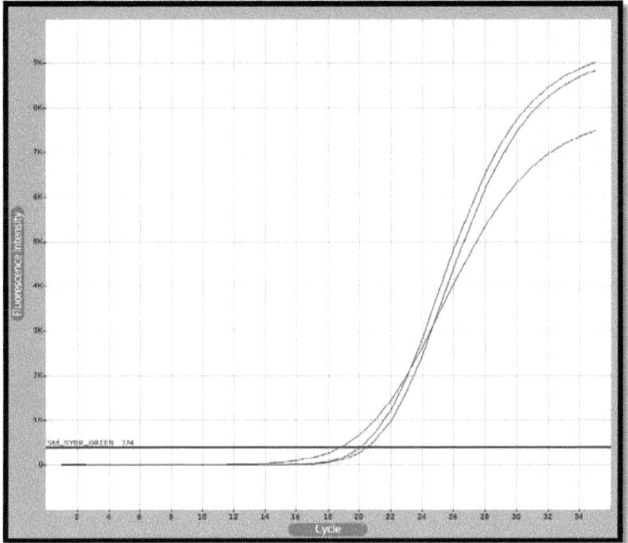

Figure (3-13, A) Amplification plot for StAR gene in the control.

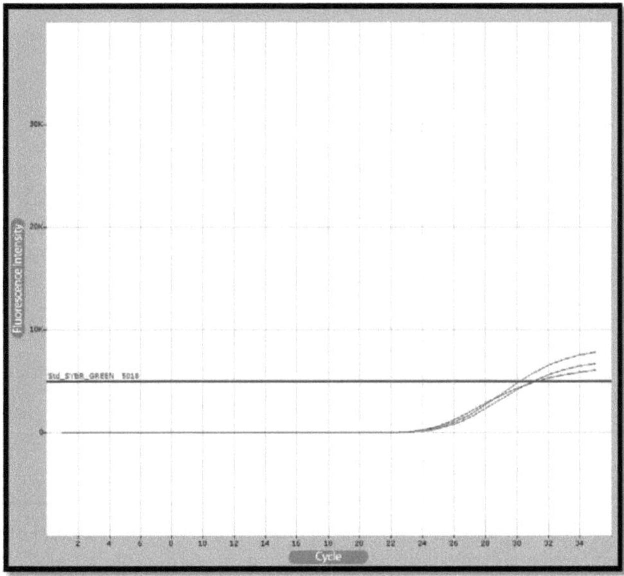

Figure (3-13, B) Amplification plot for ß-actin gene in the control

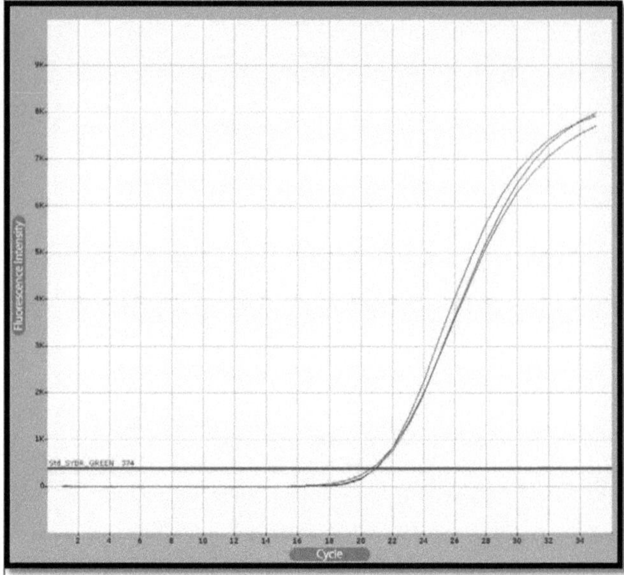

Figure (3-14, A) Amplification plot for StAR gene in 2mg/kg dose of diazepam.

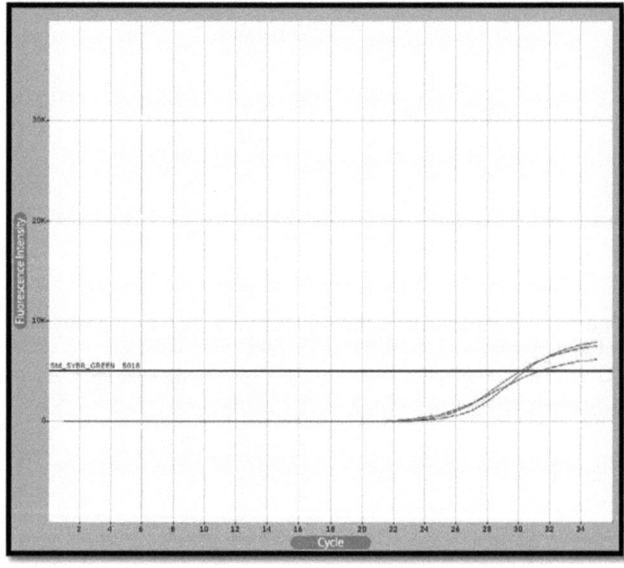

Figure (3-14,B) Amplification plot for ß-actin gene in 2mg/kg dose of diazepam.

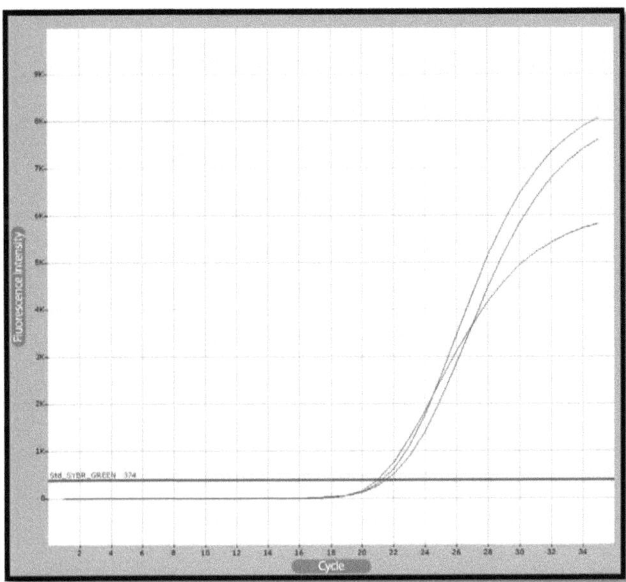

Figure (3-15, A) Amplification plot for StAR gene in 5mg/kg dose of diazepam.

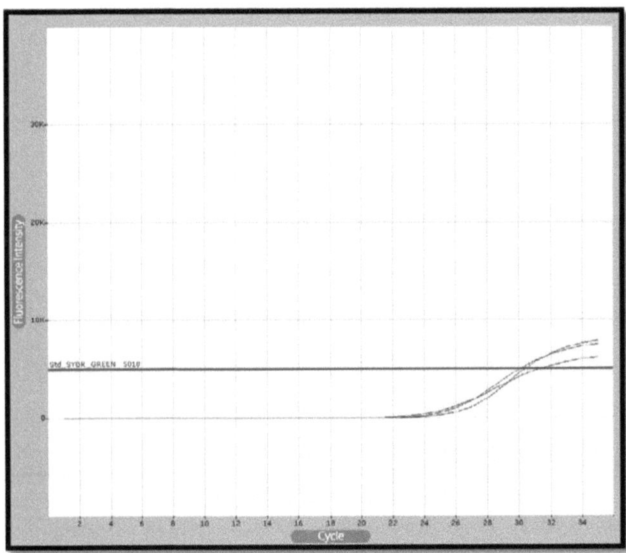

Figure (3-15, B) Amplification plot for ß-actin gene in 5mg/kg dose of diazepam.

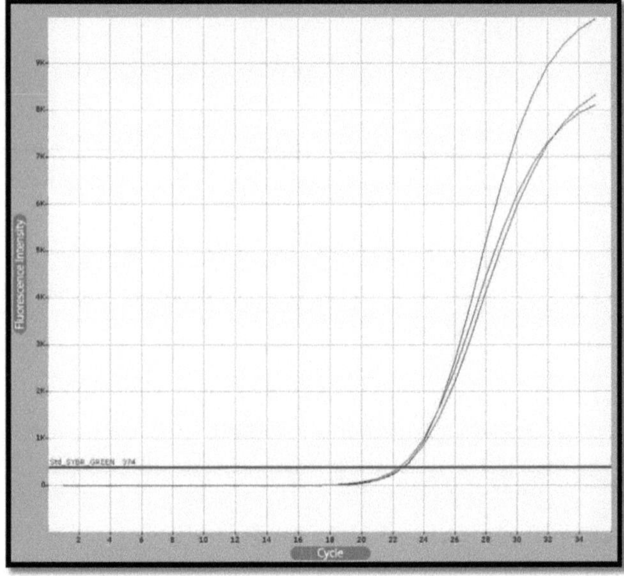

Figure (3-16,A) Amplification plot for StAR gene in 10mg/kg dose of diazepam.

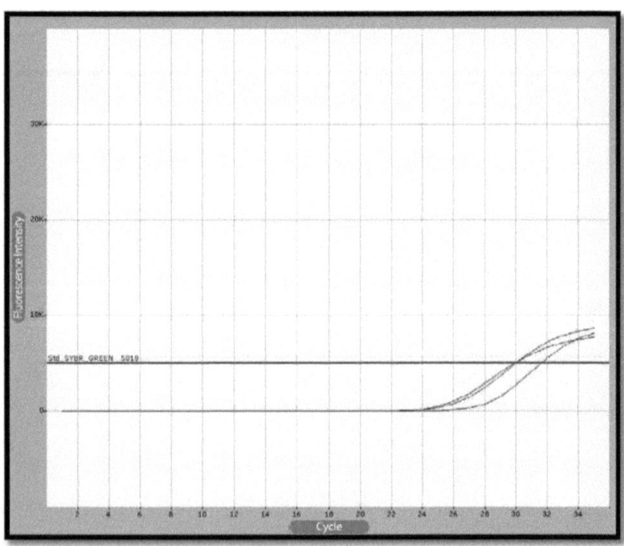

Figure (3-16, B) Amplification plot for ß-actin gene in 10mg/kg dose of
diazepam.

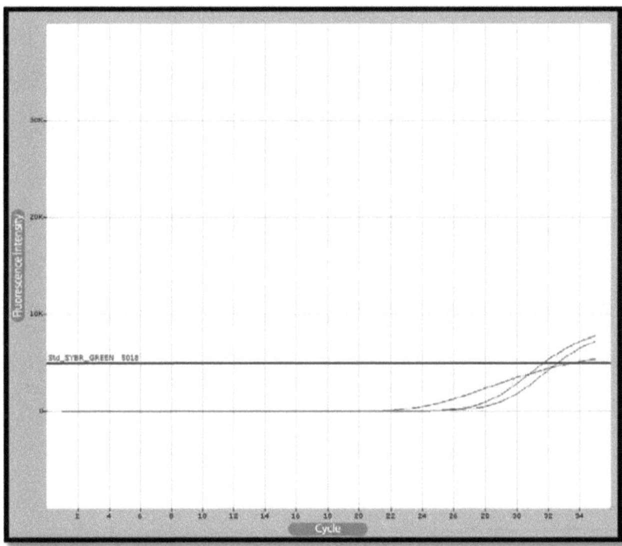

Figure (3-17, A) Amplification plot for StAR gene in sulfasalazine treatment.

Figure (3-17, B) Amplification plot for ß-actin gene in sulfasalazine treatment.

3.16 Relative gene expression:

The relative expression of the target gene (StAR) in male rats testes was calculated by using Livak method ($2^{-\triangle\triangle CT}$) that is dependent on normalization of RT-qPCR (CT values) of the target gene with housekeeping gene (ß-actin) as reference gene in control and treatment groups , table (3-6) and figure (3-18). The present results of the relative gene expression in StAR gene showed highly significant (p<0.001) difference in fold change of the gene expression levels between control and treatment groups. It showed that the relative gene expression of the StAR gene of the T2 (5mg/kg), T3 (10 mg/kg) and the sulfasalazine group; the results were (0.888±0.069; 0.66±0.038 and 0.45±0.086) respectively; were highly significantly (p<0.001)   decreased than the T1 (2mg/kg); (1.305±0.312) group. Also, the relative StAR gene expression of the T3 (10mg/kg) ;(0.66±0.038) and sulfasalazine (0.45±0.086) were significantly   (p<0.05)   decreased   than   the   T2   (5mg/kg); (0.888±0.069)group. And the relative gene expression of the sulfasalazine (0.45±0.086) group was significantly (p<0.05) decreased than the control group which is equal to 1 fold change of gene expression levels. while there was no significant difference between both the T2 (5mg/kg); (0.888±0.069) and T3 (10mg/kg);(0.66±0.038) groups compared to the control (1) group and no significant difference between the T3(10mg/kg);(0.66±0.038) and the sulfasalazine (0.45±0.086)groups.

Table (3-6) Relative gene expression between groups using RT-qPCR

Group	Control	T1(2mg/kg)	T2(5mg/kg)	T3(10mg/kg)	Sulfasalazine
Relative StAR gene expression	1	1.305±0.312	0.888±0.069 *a	0.66±0.038 *ab	0.45±0.086 *ab

Data are expressed as mean (±SE); n=3 rats/group; Values with different superscripts are significantly different.

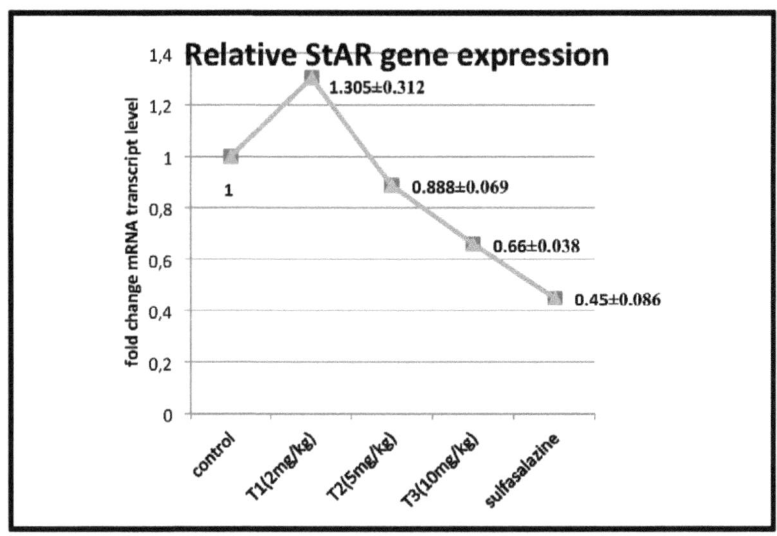

Figure (3-18) Gene expression of StAR by $2^{-\Delta\Delta CT}$ Livak method.

References

1. Agboola A. Infertility and subinfertility In Akin A., ed. Textbook of Obstetrics and Gynaecology.Vol.1, Ibadan , Heinman Educational Books,**2004**:174-76.

2. Kishore Kumar P., Raju A.B. A review on male fertility. *Hygeia. J .D Med.* **2011; 3(1)**:20-28.

3. De Kretser DM. Male infertility.*Lancet.***1997; 349:**787-90.

4. Fode M., Sonksen J., McPheeS J. and OhI D.A. Disorders of the male reproductive tract. In: McPheeeSJ, Hammer GD,eds. Pathopysiology of disease . 6th ed., New York, NY:Mc Graw-Hill,**2010**:23.

5. Costbile R.A. and Spevak M. Characterization of patients presenting with male factor infertility in an equal access, no cost medical system. *Urology* **2001;58(6)**: 1021-24.

6. Olooto W.E., Amballi A.A. and Banjo T.A. A review of female infertility; important etiological factors and management.*J Microbiol Biotechnol Res.* **2012; 2(3)**:379-85.

7. Stacey K.F. and Ryan B.D. Male infertility: An overview of the causes and treatments.*US. Pharm.* **2012; 37(6)**: 39-42.

8. Tycko.B. , Trasler JM and BestorT. Genomic imprinting: gametic mechanisms and somatic consequences. *J Androl.* **1997; 18**:480-86.

9. Pineda M. H. and Dooley M.P. McDonald s Veterinary Endocrinology and reproduction .5th ed. , Iowa state press, A Blackwell publishing company, **2003; 17(32)**:239-56.

10. Johnson M. and Everrit B.J. (eds.) Essential reproduction. Paris, Black well science Ltd. , **2000**: 212-14.

11. Romer A.S., ParsonsT. S. The Vertebrate Body. Philadelphia, PA: Holt-Saunders International. **1977**: 385–86.

12. Cunningham J.C.(ed.) Textbook of Veterinary physiology. 3rd edition, USA, Saunders company, **2002**: 421-22.

13. Toshimori K. Biology of spermatozoa maturation: an overview with an introduction to this issue. *Microscopy Research and Technique* **2003; 61(1)**:1-6

14. Molaro A., Hodges E. and Fang F. Sperm methylation profiles reveal features of epigenetic inheritance and evolution in primates. *Cell* **2011; 146:** 1029-41.

15. Surani M.A. , Barton S.C. and Norris M.L. Development of reconstituted mouse eggs suggest imprinting of the genome during gametogenesis. *Nature* **1984 ;308(5959)**:548-50.

16. Surani M.A. Evidences and consequences of differences between maternal and paternal genomes during embryogenesis in the mouse, in experimental approaches to mammalian embryonic development. In: Rossant J., Pedersen RA, Eds. Cambridge,U.K . Cambridge University press, **1986**:401-35.

17. Bartolomei M.S., Webber A.L. and Brunkow M.E. Epigenetic mechanisms underlying the imprinting of the mouse H19 gene. *Genes Dev.***1993;7(9):** 1663-73.

18. Schagdarsurengin U., Paradowska A., and Steger K. Analyzing the sperm epigenome:roles in early embryogenesis and assisted reproduction.*Nat.Rev.Urol.***2012;183**:1-11.

19. Charles M., Seiger. Fundamentals of anatomy and physiology. 4th ed Martini , Upper Saddle River, New Jersy, Prentice-Hall, **1998**:1038-55.

20. Kalthoff, K.(ed.) Analysis of biological development. Chapter 3. USA. McGraw-Hill, INC. **1996**:45-54.

21. Ohmura M., Ogawa T., Ono M., Dezawa M.,Hosaka M. and Sawada H. Increment of murine spermatogonial cell number by gonadotropin- releasing hormone analogue is independent of stem cell factor. *Biol. of Repor.***2003; 68**:2304-13.

22. Nakamoto T., Shiratsuchi A., Oda H. and Inoue K. Impaired spermatogenesis and male fertility defects in CIZ/Nmp4-disrupted mice. *J. Genes cells* **2004; 9**:575-89.

23. Fishelson L., Gon O., Holdengreber V., Delarea Y. Comparative spermatogenesis, spermatocytogenesis, and spermato-zeugmata formation in males of viviparous species of clinid fishes. The Anatomical Record: *Advances in Integrative Anatomy and Evolutionary Biology* **2007:290 (3)**: 311–23.

24. Weinbauer G.F. and Neieschlay E. Testicular physiology of primates' .In: Weinbauer GF, Korte R (eds.), Reproduction in non human primates. Munster.Waxmann.Velag.**1999:**13-26

25.Creasy D.M . Evaluation of testicular toxicity in safety evaluation studies: the appropriate use of spermatogenic staging. *Toxicol Pathol***1997; 25(2)**:122.

26. Jegou B, Pineua C, Toppan J. Assisted reproductive technology accomplishments and new horizons. Spermatogenesis in Vitro in Mammals; Cambridge, Cambridge University Press, **2002**:3–6.

27.Granner D.K. Pituitary and hypothalamic hormone. In Harper biochemistry. Murray RK, Granner DK, Mayers PA and Rodwell VW (ED), USA, Applton and Lange, **1990; 46(5)**:478-86.

28. Guyton, A.C. and Hall J.E. Textbook of medicinal physiology, Philadelphia, Pennsylvania, Elsevier Inc, **2006**:996-1006.

29. Amann R. P. Sperm production rates. In: The testis, vol. 1 (Johnson A. D., Gomes W. R., Vandemark N. L., editors.), New York, NY: Academic Press, **1970**: 433–82.

30. Kim E. B. , Susan M. B., Scott B. , Heddwen B. Ganong W.F. Review of medical physiology. 22nd edition, Toronto, New Jersy, Boston, Lange Medical books/ McGraw-Hill, **2005**: 424-30.

31. De-Rooje D.G. The effect of exogenous testosterone and estradiol on spermatogenesis multiplication in the mouse In: The testis in normal and infertile men. New York, Troen R and Nakin HR(eds.) Raven press , **1977**:85-93.

32. Vander A.J., Sheman J.H. and Luciano D.S. Reproduction In: Human physiology; the mechanism of body function.4th edithion, New York, Vender, AJ; Sheman, JH and Luciano, DS(eds.)Mc Graw- Hill book company,**1985**:551-97.

33. LeBlanc G.A., Bain L.J. and Wilson V.S. Pesticide: Multiple mechanism of demusculinization .*Mol. Cell. Endocrinol.***1997**; **126**: 1-5.

34. Calcaterra N.E. and Barrow J.C. Classics in chemical neuroscience: diazepam (valium). *ACS chemical neuroscience* **2014**; **5 (4)**: 253–60.

35. Mandrioli R., Mercolini L. and Raggi M.A. Benzodiazepine metabolism. An analytical perspective. *Curr. drug metab.* **2008**; **9 (8)**:827-44.

36. 36.Thakuria D.B. and Barthakur T. Management of musth in a male African elephant by chemical sedatives in the Assam state zoo, Guwahati. *Indian Veterinary Journal* **1996**; **73 (3)**:339-40.

37. BlažEvić N., Kajfež F. A new ring closure of 1,4-benzodiazepine. *Journal of Heterocyclic Chemistry* **1970**;**7 (5)**: 1173.

38. Zakusov V.V., Ostrovskaya R.U. and Kozhechkin S.N. Further evidence for GABA-ergic mechanisms in the action of benzodiazepines. *Internationales De Pharmacodynamie Et De Thérapie* **1977**; **229 (2)**: 313–26.

39. Riss J., Cloyd J., Gates J. and Collins S. Benzodiazepines in epilepsy: pharmacology and pharmacokinetics. *Acta Neurologica Scandinavica* **2008; 118 (2)**: 69–86.

40. Perkin, Ronald M. *Pediatric hospital medicine : textbook of inpatient management* (2nd ed.). Philadelphia: Wolters Kluwer Health/Lippincott Williams & Wilkins.**2008; 862.**

41. Vozeh S. Pharmacokinetic of benzodiazepines in old age *.Schweizerische Medizinische Wochenschrift* **1981;111 (47)**: 1789–93.

42. Cardauns H. and Iffland R . Fatal intoxication of a young drug addict with diazepam. *Arch Toxicol* **1973; 31:** 147-151.

43. Clark G.C. Isolation and identification of drugs, 1st ed. London, William Clowes, **1978**:870.

44. Ballenger J.C. Benzodiazepine receptors agonists and antagonists. In Sadock VA, Sadock BJ, Kaplan HI (eds.). Kaplan and Sadock's Comprehensive Textbook of Psychiatry, 7th ed., Lippincott Williams & Wilkins. **2000**:2317–23.

45. Rapoport M.J., Lanctôt K.L., Streiner D.L., Bédard M., Vingilis E., Murray B., Schaffer A., Shulman K.I. and Herrmann N. Benzodiazepine use and driving: a meta-analysis. *J Clin Psychiatry* **2009; 70 (5)**: 663–73.

46. Orriols L., Salmi L.R., Philip P., Moore N., Delorme B., Castot A.and Lagarde E. The impact of medicinal drugs on traffic safety: a systematic review of epidemiological studies . *Pharmacoepidemiol Drug Saf* **2009; 18 (8)**: 647–58.

47. Horimoto M., Isobe Y., Isogai Y., Tachibana M. Rat epididimal sperm motion changes induced by ethylene glycol monoethyl ether, sulfasalazine and 2,5-hexandione. *Reprod Toxicol* **2000;14**:55–63.

48. Virginia A.B, Victoria Linares A.B., Montserrat Bellés a,b, Maria L. Albinaa,b, Juan J. Sirvent c, José L. Domingoa,*, Domènec J. Sánchez a,b. Sulfasalazine induced oxidative stress: A possible mechanism of male infertility . *Reproductive Toxicology* **2009;27**: 35–40 .

49. Steele G.L., Leung P.C. Intragonadal signalling mechanisms in the control of steroid hormone production. *J Steroid Biochem Mol Biol* **1992; 41:** 515–22.

50. Li L.H., Wine R.N., Miller D.S., Reece J.M. and Smith M. Protection against methoxyacetic-acid-induced spermatocyte apoptosis with calcium channel blockers in cultured rat seminiferous tubules: possible mechanisms. *Toxicol Appl Pharmacol* **1997; 144:** 105–19.

51. Publicover S.J., Barratt C.L. Voltage-operated Ca2+ channels and the acrosome reaction: which channels are present and what do they do? *Hum Reprod* **1999; 14:** 873–9.

52. Berridge MJ, Lipp P, Bootman MD. The versatility and universality of calcium signalling. *Nat Rev Mol Cell Biol* **2000; 1:** 11–21.

53. Rommerts F.F., Lyng F.M., von Ledebur E., Quinlan L. and Jones G.R. Calcium confusion-is the variability in calcium response by Sertoli cells to specific hormones meaningful or simply redundant? *J Endocrinol* **2000; 167:** 1–5.

54. Rossato M., Nogara A., Merico M., Ferlin A. and Garolla A. Store-operated calcium influx and stimulation of steroidogenesis in rat Leydig cells: role of Ca^{2+} activated K^+ channels. *Endocrinology* **2001; 142:** 3865–72.

55. Machaca K. Ca^{2+} calmodulin-dependent protein kinase II potentiates store-operated Ca^{2+} current. *J Biol Chem* **2003; 278**: 33730–7.

56. Bergh JJ, Xu Y, Farach-Carson MC. Osteoprotegerin expression and secretion are regulated by calcium influx through the L-type voltage-sensitive calcium channel. *Endocrinology* **2004; 145**: 426–36.

57. Yamaguchi M. Role of regucalcin in maintaining cell homeostasis and function. *Int J Mol Med* **2005; 15:** 371–89.

58. Barrat C.L., Publicover S.J. Interaction between sperm and zona pellucida in male fertility. *Lancet* **2001;358**:1660-2.

59. Hille B. Calcium channels. In: Hille B, ed. Ionic Channels of Excitable Membranes, 2nd edition,. Sunderland, MA: Sinauer, **1992**:83.

60. Sullivan M.H. and Cooke B.A. The role of Ca^{2+} steroidogenesis in Leydig cells: stimulation of intracellular free Ca^{2+} by lutropin (LH), luliberin (LHRH) agonist and cyclic AMP. *Biochem J* **1986; 236**: 45–51.

61. Tomić M, Dufau ML, Catt KJ, Stojilkovic SS. Calcium signalling in single rat Leydig cells. *Endocrinology* **1995; 136**: 3422–29.

62. Adebanjo OA, Igietseme J, Huang CL, Zaidi M. The effect of extracellularly applied divalent cations on cytosolic Ca2+ in murine Leydig cells: evidence for a Ca2+-sensing receptor. *J Physiol* **1998; 513:** 399–410.

63. Kawa K. Existence of calcium channels and intercellular coupling in the testosterone-secreting cells of the mouse. *J Physiol* **1987; 393**: 647–66.

64. Arnoult C., Villaz M., Florman H.M. Pharmacological properties of the T-type Ca^{2+} current of mouse spermatogenic cells. *Mol Pharmacol* **1998**; **53**: 1104–11.

65. Costa RR, Varanda WA. Intracellular calcium changes in mice Leydig cells are dependent on calcium entry through T-type calcium channels. *J Physiol* **2007**; **585**: 339–49.

66. Breitbart H. Intracellular calcium regulation in sperm capacitation and acrosomal reaction. *Mol Cell Endocrinol* **2002**; **187**:139-44.

67. Kirkman-Brown J.C., Punt E.L, Barrat CL. and Publicover S.J .Zona Pellucida and progesterone-induced Ca^{2+} signaling and acrosome reaction in human spermatozoa. *J Androl* **2002**; **23**:306-15.

68. Nikpoor B., Mowla S.J.Movaheden M. and Ziaee S.A. Cat sper gene expression in postnatal development of mouse testes and subfertile men with deficient sperm motility. *Hum Reprod* **2004**; **19**:124-8.

69. Suarez S.S., Ho H.C . Hyperactivatedmotility in sperm. *Reprod Domest Anim* **2003**; **38**:119-24.

70. Matlib M.A., Schwartz A. Selective effects of diltiazem, a benzothiazepine calcium channel blocker, and diazepam, and other benzodiazepines on the Na+/ Ca2+ exchange carrier system of heart and brain mitochondria. *Life Sci.***1983**; **32(25)**:2837-42.

71. William C.T. and DeLorenzo R.J. Micromolar-affinity benzodiazepine receptors regulate voltage-sensitive calcium channels in nerve terminal preparations . *Proceedings of the National Academy of Sciences of the United States of America* **1984; 81 (10)**: 3118–22.

72. Hullihan J. P., Spector S., Taniguchi T. and Wang J. K. The binding of [3H]-diazepam to guinea-pig ileal longitudinal muscle

and the in vitro inhibition of contraction by benzodiazepines. *Br. J. Pharmacol.***1983; 78:** 321-27.

73. Syapin,P.J. and Skolnick, P. Characterization of benzodiazepine binding sites in cultured cells of neural origin. *J. Neurochem.***1979; 32:** 1047- 51.

74. Wang J. K. , Morgan J. I. and Spector S. *Fed. Proc. Fed. Am. Soc. Exp. Biol.***1982; 41:** 1328.

75.Schaufele P., Schumacher E. , Acevedo C.G. and Contreras E. Diazepam, adenosine analogues and calcium channel antagonists inhibit the contractile activity of the mouse urinary bladder. *Arch Int pharmacodyn Ther.***1995; 329(3):** 454-66.

76.Dufau M.L. Endocrine regulation and communicating functions of the Leydig cell. *Ann Rev Physiol* **1988; 50:** 483–508.

77. Saez J.M. Leydig cells: endocrine, paracrine, and autocrine regulation. *Endocr Rev* **1994; 15:** 574–626.

78. Chen Y.C., Nagpal M.L., Stocco D.M. and Lin T. Effects of genistein, resveratrol, and quercetin on steroidogenesis and proliferation of MA-10 mouse Leydig tumor cells. *J Endocrinol* **2007; 192:** 527–37.

79.Merelli F., Stojilkovic S., Lida T. and Catt K.J.Gonadotropin-releasing hormone induced calcium signaling in clonal pituitary gonadotrops. *Endocrinology* **1992;131:**925-32.

80.Sriraman V., Sairman M.R. and Rao A.J. Evaluation of relative role of LH and FSH in regulation of differentiation of Leydig cells using EDS treated adult rat model. *J Endocrinol* **2003;176:**151-61.

81. Saez J.M., Lejeune H. Regulation of Leydig cell functions by hormones and growth factors other than LH and IGF-1. In: Payne A.H., Hardy M.P., Russell L.D. (Eds.). The Leydig cell. Vienna, Cache River Press, **1996** IL:383-406.

82. Medelson C., Dufau M.L., Catt K.J. Gonadotropin binding and stimulation of cAMP and testosterone production in isolated Leydig cells. *J Biol Chem* **1975; 250**: 8818–23.

83. Gorczynska-Fjalling E. The role of calcium in signal transduction processes in sertoli cells. *Reprod Biol* **2004; 4**:219-41.

84. Manna P.R., Pakarinen P., El-Hefnawy T. and Huhtaniemi I.T. Functional assessment of the calcium messenger system in cultured mouse Leydig tumor cells: regulation of human chorionic gonadotropin induced expression of the steroidogenicacute regulatory protein. *Endocrinology* **1999;140**:1739-51.

85. Ma X.H., Shi Y.L.,Sheng L.i. A patch clamp study on reconsistituted calcium permeable channels of human sperm plasma membranes. *Sheng Li Xue Bao***1999;51**:571-9.

86. Gou B. The sertoli cells. *Baillier 's Clin Endocrinol Metabol* **1992;6**:273-311.

87. Griswold M.D. Action of FSH on mammalian sertoli cells. In: The sertoli cells, L.D. Russel & M.D Griswold eds. Cache River Press. Clearwater F.L, **1993**:493-509.

88. Means A.R, Dedman J.R., Tash J.S. and Tindell D.J. Regulation of the testis sertoli cells by follicle stimulating hormone. *Annu Rev Physiol* **1980;42**:59-70.

89. Benton L., Shan L.X. and Hardey M.P. Differentiation of adult Leydig cells. *J steroid Biochem Mol.Biol.* **1995;53**:61-68.

90. Walker W.H., Cheng J. FSH and testosterone signaling in Sertoli cells. *Reproduction* **2005;130**:15-28.

91. Arnoult C., Cardullo R.A. ,Lemos J.R. and Florman H.M. Activation of mouse sperm T-type calcium channels by adhesion to the egg zona pellucid . *Proc Natl Acad Sci USA*.**1996;93**:13004-13009.

92. De La Vega-Beltran JL, Sánchez-Cárdenas C, Krapf D, Hernandez-González EO, Wertheimer E, Treviño CL, Visconti PE, Darszon A. Mouse sperm membrane potential hyperpolarization is necessary and sufficient to prepare sperm for the acrosome reaction. *J Biol Chem.* **2012** ;**287(53)**:44384-93.

93. Komura H. and Rakic P. Intracellular calcium fluctuations modulate the rate of neuronal migration, *Neuron* **1996;17**:275-85.

94. Arnoult C., Kazam I.G.,Visconti P.E, Kopf G.S. and Florman H.M. Control of the low voltage-activated calcium channel of mouse sperm by egg ZP3 and by membrane hyperpolirization during capacitation. *Proc Natl Acad Sci USA.***1999;96**:6757-62.

95. Arnoult C., Cardullo R.A. ,Lemos J.R. and Florman H.M. Activation of mouse sperm T-type calcium channels by adhesion to the egg zona pellucid . *Proc Natl Acad Sci USA.***1996;93**:13004-13009.

96. Westenbroek R.E, Babcock D.F. Discrete regional distributions suggest diverse functional roles of calcium channels alpha1 subunits in sperms. *Dev Biol* **1999;207**:457-469.

97. Yanagimachi R. Requirement of extracellular calcium ions for various stages of fertilization and fertilization- related phenomena in the hamster. *Gamate Res.***1982; 5**:323-44.

98. Suarez S.S.,Vincenti L.,Ceglia M.W. Hyperactivated motility induced in mouse sperm by calcium ionophore A23187 is reversible .*J Exp Zool* **1987;244**:331-36.

99. Swerdloff R.S. and Wang C. The testis and male sexual function. In: Goldman L. ,Ausiello D. (eds.) Cecil Textbook of Medicine, 22nd edition, Philadelphia, P.A.:W.B.Saunders, **2004**:1472-83.

100. Swerdloff, R. S.; Wang, C. and Hikim, A. P. S. Hypothalamic –pituitary –gonodal axis in men In:Hormones ,beain

and behavier .Pfaff, Q. W. d. Springer-verlagBerlin Heiderberg, New York. **2010** : 1-8.

101. Lane K. Christenson, Jerome F. Strauss III. Steroidogenic acute regulatory protein(StAR) and the intramitochondrial translocation of cholesterol. *Biochemica et Biophsica Acta* **2000; 1529**:175-87.

102. Hannas BR, Lambright CS, Furr J, Evans N, Foster PMD, Gray EL, Wilson VS. Genomic biomarkers of phthalate-induced male reproductive developmental toxicity: A targeted RT-PCR array approach for defining relative potency. *Toxicological Sciences* **2012; 125(2)**:544-557.

103. Orme-Johnson N.R., Epstein L.F and Alberta J.A. Mitochondrial localization of a phosphoprotein that rapidly accumulates in adrenal cortex cells exposed to adrenocorticotropic hormone or to CAMP. *J Biol. Chem* **1989; 264**: 2368-72.

104. Saiki R.K., Gelfand D.H. , Stofell S., Scharf S.J., Higuchi R., Horn G.T.,Mullis K.B. and Erlich H.A. . Primer directed enzymatic amplification of DNA with a thermostable DNA polymerase. *Science* **1988; 239**:487-91.

105. Simpson E.R. and Boyd G.S. The cholesterol side- chain cleavage system of the adrenal cortex: a mixed function oxidase. *Biochem. Biophys. Res. Commun.***1966; 24**:10-17.

106. Steven R King, Douglas M Stocco. Steroidogenic Acute Regulatory Protein Expression in the Central Nervous System. *Front Endocrinol (Lausanne)* **2011; 2(72)**:1-6.

107. Mary Cherian-Shaw, Muraly Puttabyatappa, Erin Greason, Annabelle Rodriguez, Catherine A. VandeVoort, and Charles L. Chaffin. Expression of Scavenger Receptor-BI and Low-Density Lipoprotein Receptor and Differential Use of Lipoproteins to

Support Early Steroidogenesis in Luteinizing Macaque Granulosa Cells. *Endocrinology* **2009 ; 150(2)**: 957–65.

108.	Papadopoulos V, Baraldi M, Guilarte TR, Knudsen TB, Lacapère JJ, Lindemann P, Norenberg MD, Nutt D, Weizman A, Zhang MR, Gavish M. Translocator protein (18kDa): new nomenclature for the peripheral-type benzodiazepine receptor based on its structure and molecular function. *Trends Pharmacol Sci.* **2006;27(8)**:402-9.

109.	Kanako Morohaku, Susanne H. Pelton, Daniel J. Daugherty, W. Ronald Butler,Wenbin Deng, and Vimal Selvaraj. Translocator Protein/Peripheral Benzodiazepine Receptor Is Not Required for Steroid Hormone Biosynthesis. *Endocrinology* **2014; 155(1)**:89–97.

110.	Stocco D.M. StAR protein and the regulation of steroid hormone biosynthesis. *Annual review of physiology* **2001; 63:** 193–213.

111.	Strom JG Jr, Kalu AU. Formulation and stability of diazepam suspension compounded from tablets. *Am J Hosp Pharm.* **1986 ;43(6)**:1489-91.

112.	Zita Szalai, Krisztina Kupai, Médea Veszelka, Anikó Pósa, Szilvia Török Anikó Magyariné Berkó, Zoltán Baráth, Ferenc A. Lászl, Csaba Varga. Novel features of the rat model of inflammatory bowel disease based on 2,4,6 trinitrobenzenesulfonic acid-induced acute colitis. *Acta Biologica Szegediensis* **2014; 58(2)**:127-132.

113.	Chaloob, Rasool; Numan, Intisar Tarik; Taher, Mohammed Abbas. Effect of nimodipine on steroidogenesis in male rats. *International Journal of Science & Nature* **2013; 4(1)**:150-55.

114. Saadat Parhizkar, Maryam Jamielah Yusoff, and Mohammad Aziz Dollah . Effect of Phaleria macrocarpa on sperm characteristics in adult rats. *Advanced pharmaceutical Bulletin* **2013; 3(2)**:345-52.

115. Fey, P., Kowal, A. S., Gaudet, P., Pilcher, K. E., Chisholm, R. L. Protocols for growth and development of Dictyostelium discoideum. *Nat Protoc* **2007; 2**:1307-16

116. Chemineau P., Cogine Y. , Guerin Y. , Orgeure P. and Valtet J.C. Training Manual on Artificial Insemination in sheep and goats. FAO, Animal Production and Health **1991:** 83.

117. Siegmund O.H. (ed.) Reproductive and urinary system. In: Merk Veterinary manual. Siegmund O.H. and Fraser C.M . USA, Merck and co. Inc. Rahway N.J., **1979**:794-890.

118. Cumming, D.C., Vickovic, M.W., Wall, S.R. and Fluker, M.R. Defects in pulsatile LH release in normally menstruating runners. *J. Clin. Endocrinol. Metab.***1985; 60:** 810–12.

119. Carl A.B., Edward R.A., David E.B. (eds.).Tietz textbook of Clinical chemistry and molecular Diagnosics. 5th ed. Chapter 50. Pituitary function, Philadelphia, Hsevier Saunders Co,**2012** :1970-2000.

120. KleeGG, Heser DW. Techniques to measure testosterone in the elderly. *Myo Clin Proc* **2000;75** Suppl :519-25.

121. Ratnasooriya WD, Jayakody JRAC, Premakumara GAS. Adverse pregnancy outcome in rats following exposure to a Salacia reticulata (Celastracea) root extract. *Braz J Med Biol Res.***2003;36**:931–935.

122.   Luna L.G. (ed.). Manual of histology staining. Methods of armed forces Institute of pathology. 3rd edition, New York and London, McGraw-Hill Book Company, **1968**.

123.   Bancroft J. and Stevens A. (eds.). Theory and practice of Histological techniques, 2nd edition. Edinburgh ; New York : Churchill Livingstone. . **1982**:624.

124.   Sanaz Dastgheib, Cambyz Irajie, Raheleh Assaei, Farhad Koohpeima, and Pooneh Mokarram. Optimization of RNA Extraction from Rat Pancreatic Tissue. *Iran J Med Sci.* **2014** ; **39(3)**: 282–88.

125.   Okamoto T, Okabe S.Ultraviolet absorbance at 260 and 280 nm in RNA measurement is dependent on measurement solution. *Int J Mol Med.* **2000** ;**5(6)**:657-9.

126.   Joyce C. Quantitative RT-PCR. A review of current methodologies. *Methods Mol. Biol. **2002;193**: 83–92.*

127.   Harisha S: Biotechnology procedures and experiments handbook. Infinity science press LLC, New Delhi, India **2007**:121-23.

128.   Lee P.Y., Costumbrado J. and Hsu C.Y. Agarose gel electrophoresis for the separation of DNA fragements. *J.Vis.Exp* **2012**:3923.

129.   Robinson D.H. and Lafleche G.L.: nucleic acid electrophoresis in agarose gel .Essential Molecular Biology, 2nd edition, Oxford University Press, TA Brawn, **2000; 1**:5.

130.   Saiki, R.K., Gelfand, D.H., Stoffel, S., Scharf , S.J., Higuchi, R., Horn, G.T., Mullis, K.B. and Erlich, H.A., 1988. Primer-directed enzymatic amplification of DNA with a thermostable DNA polymerase. *Science***1988; 239**:487–91.

131. Livak, K.J., Schmittgen, T.D. Analysis of relative gene expression data using real- time quantitative PCR and the 2 (-Delta Delta CT) method. *Methods* **2001; 25**:402-10.

132. Ruth Ravid. Practical statistics for educators. In: 4th edition. Rowman and Littlefield publishers, Lanham, Maryland ,united Kigdom, part 5, inferential statistics, **2011**:143-187.

133. Chowdhury M. and Steinberger E. Differences of the effects of testosterone propionate on the production of LH and FSH. *Act. Endocinologica* **1976; 82**:688-90.

134. Reddy C.M., Murthy D.R. and Patil S.B. Antispermatogenic and androgenic activities of various extracts of Hibiscus rosa sinensis in albino mice. *Ind.J.Exp.Biol.***1997; 35**:1170-74.

135. Nassem M.Z. , Patil S.R. and Patil S.B. Antispermatogenic antiandrogenic activities of Momordica charantia (Karela) in albino rats. *J.Ethnopharmacol.* **1998; 61**:9-16.

136. Cook P.S., Notelovitz M.and Kalra S.P. Effect of diazepam on serum testosterone and the ventral prostate gland in male rats. *Arch Androl* **1979; 3(1)**:31-5.

137. O'Shaughnessy P. J. , Monteiro A., Verhoeven G., De Gendt K. and Abel M.H. Effect of FSH on testicular morphology and spermatogenesis in gonadotrophin-deficient hypogonadal mice lacking androgen receptors. *Reproduction.* **2010 ; 139(1)**: 177–184.

138. Naor Z. and Catt K.J. mechanism of action of gonadotropin releasing hormone. Involvement of phospholipids turnover in luteinizing hormone release. *J. Biol. Chem.***1981; 256**: 2226-29.

139. Chubb C. Genes regulating testes size. *Biol.Reprt.***1992; 47**: 29-36.

140. Steinberger E. Hormonal control of mammalian spermatogenesis. *Physiological Reviews* **1971; 51**:1-22.

141. Black H.E., Szot R.J., Arthaud L.E., Massa T., Mylecraine L., Klein M., Lake R., Fabry A., Kaminska G.Z., SinhaD. P., et al. Preclinical safty evaluation of the benzodiazepine quazepam. *Arzneimittelforsechung* **1987;37(8)**:906-13.

142. Gulati D., Grimes L., Barnes L. Reproductive toxicology . Diazepam. *Environ Health Perspect* **1997;105(1)**:297-98.

143. Swerdloff R. and Glass A.R. Male Reproductive abnormalities Chapter 7.In: Endocrine pathophysiology. A patient oriented approch. Hershman J.M.(ed), Philadeliphia, Lea and Febiger ,**1977:**177.

144. Behre H.M., Nashan D., Hubert W. and Nieschlag E. Gonadotropin releasing hormone agonist blunts the androgen induced suppression of spermatogenesis in a clinical trial of male contraception. *Journal of Clinical Endocrinology and metabolism* **1992; 74(1)**: 84-90.

145. Christensen A.C . Leydig cell: In: Handbook of physiology, P.O. Greep and E.B. Astwood. Washington DC American physiological Society.**1975**:165-172.

146. Baldessarini R.J. Indrugs and the treatment of psychiatric disorders. The pharmacological basis of therapeutics Ed. By Goodman and Gilman. Macmillan Pub.Co.Inc.**1980**:301-417.

147. Bloom W. and Fawcett D.W. Male reproductive system. In the textbook of Histology, Saunders company, Philadelphia, **1975**.

148. Cooper T.G. The epididymis as a site of contraceptive attack. In: spermatogenesis fertilization, contraception, Nieschlag E. and Habenicbt U.F. (Eds.), Berlin, Springer, **1992**: 419-60.

149. Lohiya N.K. Goyal R.B, Jayaprakash, D.;Sharma, S.;Kumer M. and Ansari, A.S. Introduction of reversible antifertility with a crude ethanol extract of Carica papya seeds in albino male rats. *Int.J. Pharmacognosy* **1992; 30**: 308-20.

150. Gupat G., Srivastava A.K. and Setty B.S. Androgenic regulation of glycoltic and HMP pathway in epididymis and vas deferens of rhesus monkey. *Ind.J.Exp.Biol.* **1993; 31**:305-11.

151. Ansari A.S., Kumar S., Srivastava S. and Lohiya N.K. Longterm sequelae of tolnidamine on male reproduction and general body metabolism in rabbits. *Contraception* **1998; 57**:271-79.

152. Hou J.W., Collins D.C, and Schliecher R.L Source of cholesterol for testosterone biosynthesis in murine Leydig cells. *Endocrinology.* **1990;127(5)**:2047-55.

153. Ruffoli R. A., Carpi M. A. ,Giambelluca L. Grasso M. C. Scavuzzo and Giannessi F._Diazepam administration prevents testosterone decrease and lipofuscin accumulation in testis of mouse exposed to chronic noise stress. *Andrologia* **2006;38(5)**:159–65.

154. Meena R., Misro M.M., Ghosh D. and Nandan D. Extended intervention time and evaluation of sperm suppression by dienogest plus testosterone undecanoate in male rat. *Contraception* **2012; 85(1)**:113-21.

155. Kato M., Makino S., Kimura H. and Hirano K. In vitro evaluation of acrosomal status and motility in rat epididymal spermatozoa treated with a-chlorohydrin for predicting their fertilizing capacity .*J. Reprod.Develop*$^{2+}$.**2002;48**:461-68.

156. Ohashi K., Saji F., Kato M. and Tomiyama T. Acrobeads test : A new diagnostic test for assessment of the fertilizing capacity of human spermatozoa. *Fertil. Steril.***1995; 63**:625-30.

157. Mohana K.M., Asha K. and Mathura P.P. Diazepam: a peripheral benzodiazepines receptor ligand, inhibits mitochondrial F1-F0 ATPase and induces oxidative stress in goat epididymal sperm in vitro. *International journal of Scientific and engineering research* **2013; 4(8)**:1963-69.

158. Bowman W.C. and Rand M.J. (eds.) The reproductive system and drugs affecting the reproductive systems. Textbook of pharmacology, 2nd edition, **1985; 20**:1-8.

159. William K.W. Hormones and hormone antagonists. Alfonso R.G. In: Remington, The Science and Practice of pharmacy, 20th edition, vol 11, **2000; 77**: 1390-91.

160. Kar R.N. and Das R.K. Induction of sperm head abnormalities in mice by three tranquilizers. *Cytobio.* **1983; 36(141)**:45-51.

161. Tamio F., Masashi K., Tetsuya A., Yoshimasa H. and Masao H. Effects of sulfasalazine on sperms acrosome reaction and gene expression in the male reproductive organs of rats, *Toxicological Sciences* **2005; 85**: 675-682.

162. Pakarainen T., Zhang F., Makela S. and Huhtaniemi I. Testosterone replacement therapy induces spermatogenesis and partially restore fertility in luteinizing hormone receptor Knockout mice. *Endocrinology* **2005; 146(2)**:596-606.

163. Guillete L.J., Pickford D.B., Crain D.A. and Percival H.F. Reduction in penis size and plasma testosterone concentration in juvenile alligators living in a contaminated environment. *Gen. and Comp.Endocrine.* **1996;101**:32-42.

164. Einstein R., Jones R.S., Knifton A. and Srarmer G.A. Principles of veterinary therapeutics. Singapore, Longman Scientific and technical. **1994**: 288-89.

165. Calvo D.J., Campos M.B., Calandra R.S., Medina J.H.., Ritta M.N. Effect of long term diazepam administration on testicular benzodiazepine receptors and steroidogenesis. *Life Sci* **1991;49(7)**: 519-25.

166. Chaudhary R., Ashish R.S. and Mali P.C. Reversible contraceptive efficacy and safety evaluation of ethanolic extract of Maytenus emargineta in male albino rats. *Journal of pharmacy research* **2011; 4(1)**:213-16.

167. Cuparencu B, Tomus C, Horák J, Nan A, Cordos M, Puia L, Scafuro MA, Marmo E. Effects of the intraperitoneal administration of diazepam on rat serum lipoproteins separated by polyacrylamide gel electrophoresis. *Clin Exp Pharmacol Physiol.* **1985;12(6)**:593-602.

168. Prasad M.R and Rajalakshmi M. Spermatogenesis and accessory gland secretions. In: Textbook of biochemistry and human biology. 2nd edition, India private limited , New Delhi, Talwar G.P., Srivastava L.M. and Moudgil L.M. Eds., Prentice-Hallof ,**1989**:883.

169. Payne A. H., and Hales D. B. Overview of steroidogenic enzymes in the pathway from cholesterol to active steroid hormones. *Endocr. Rev.* **2004; 25**: 947–70.

170. Barlow N. J., Phillips, S. L., Wallace D. G., Sar M., Gaido K. W., and Foster P. M. Quantitative changes in gene expression in fetal rat testes following exposure to di(n-butyl) phthalate. *Toxicol. Sci.* **2003; 73**: 431–41.

171.   Cao G., Zhao L., Stangl H., Hasegawa T., Richardson J. A., Parker K. L. and Hobbs H. H. Developmental and hormonal regulation of murine scavenger receptor, class B, type 1. *Mol. Endocrinol.* **1999; 13**: 1460–73.

172.   Bourguignon J.P., Gerard A., Rose J .and Franchimont P. Pulstile release of GnRH from the rat hypothalamus in vitro: calcium and glucose dependency and inhibition by superactive GnRH analogs. *Endocrinology* **1987; 121**:993-99.

173.   Haisenlader D.J. Ferris H.A. and Shupnik M.A. The calcium component of gonadotropins releasing hormone stimulated luteinizing hormone subunit gene transcription is mediated by calcium- calmodulin dependent protein kinase type II. *Endocrinology* **2008;149**:3330-38.

174.   Rai J., Pandey S.N., Srivastava R.K. Testosterone hormone level in albino rats following restraint stress of long duration. *J.Anat.Soc.India* **2004; 53 (1)**:17-19 .

175.   Noar Z. and Catt K.J. Mechanism of action of gonadotropin releasing hormone. Involvement of phospholipids turnover in lutenizing hormone release. *J.Biol.Chem.***1981;256**:2226-29.

176.   Leong D.A. and Thorner M.O. A potential code of lutenizing hormone releasing hormone induced calicium ion responses in the regulation of luteinizing hormone secretion among individual gonadotropes. *J. Biol. Chem.* **1991;266**:9016-22.

177.   Thomas P., Mellon P.L., Turgeon J.L. and Waring D.W. The L beta T2 clonal gonadotrope: a model of single cell studies of endocrine cell secretion. *Endocrinology* **1996;137**:2979-89.

178.   Smith C.E., Wakefield I., King J.S. The initial phase of GnRH stimulated LH release from pituitary cells is independent of

calcium entry through voltage gated channels. *FEBS Lett.* **1987;225**:247-50.

179. Leong D.A. and Thorner M.O.A potential code of Luteinizing hormone- releasing hormone induced calcium ion responses in the regulation of Luteinizing hormone secretion among individual gonadotropes. *J.Biol.Chem* **1991; 266**: 9016-22.

180. Garner D.L. and Hafez E.S. Spermatozoa and seminal plasma . In Hafez ES (eds.) Reproduction in farm animals. 6th edition, Philadeliphia., USA, Lea and Febiger, **1993**:165-87.

181. Liu D.Y. and Baker H.W. Tests of human sperm function and fertilization in vitro. *Fertil. Steril.* **1992;58**:465-483.

182. Mahadevan M.M. and Trounson A.O. The influence of seminal characteristics on the success rate of human in vitro fertilization . *Fertil. Steril.* **1984; 42**: 400-5.

183. Guerriero F.J., Fox K.A. Benzodiazepines and reproduction of Swiss-Webster mice. *Res Commun Chem Pathol Pharmacol* **1976; 13(4)**: 601-10.

184. Hess R.A., Linder R.E., Strader L.F. and Perreault S.D. Acute effects and long-term sequelae of 1,3 dinitrobenzene on male reproduction in the rat. II Quantitative and qualitative histopathology of the testes. *J Androl.***1988; 5**:327-42.

185. Hall P.F . Testicular steroid synthesis: organization and regulation. In: physiology of reproduction. Eds: Knobil E., Neill JD., New York, Raven Press, **1994; 1**:1335-62.

186. Jeyakumar M.,Suresh R., Krishnamurthy H.N. and Moudgal N.R. Changes in testicular function following specific deprivation of LH in the adult male rabbit. *J Endocrinol.* **1995; 147**:111-20.

187. Nair N.; Bedwal R.S. and Mathur R.S. Effect of adrenalactomy and hydrocortisone treatment on histopathological , biochemical and zinc and copper profiles in rat testes . *Indian J Expt Biol.* **1995; 33**:655-63.

188. Ritzen E.M., Boitani C. and Parvinen M. Cyclic secretion of protein by the rat seminiferous tubules depending on the stage of spermatogenesis. *Int J Androl* (Suppl.) **1981; 3**: 57-8.

189. Hasegawa, T., Zhao, L., Caron, K. M., Majdic, G., Suzuki, T., Shizawa, S., Sasano, H., and Parker, K. L. Developmental roles of the steroidogenic acute regulatory protein (StAR) as revealed by StAR knockout mice. *Mol. Endocrinol.* **2000; 14**: 1462–71.

190. Manna P. R., Roy P., Clark B. J., Stocco D. M., and Huhtaniemi I. T. Interaction of thyroid hormone and steroidogenic acute regulatory (StAR) protein in the regulation of murine Leydig cell steroidogenesis. *J. Steroid Biochem. Mol. Biol.* **2001; 76**: 167–77.

191. Clark B. J., Soo S. C., Caron K. M., Ikeda Y., Parker K. L., and Stocco D. M. Hormonal and developmental regulation of the steroidogenic acute regulatory protein. *Mol. Endocrinol.* **1995; 9**: 1346–55.

192. Stocco D. M. and Clark B.J. Regulation of the acute production of steroids in steroidogenic cells. *Endocr. Rev.* **1996; 17**: 221–44.

193. Hall P.F., Osawa S. and Mrotek J. The influence of calmodulin on steroid synthesis in Leydig cells from rat testis. *Endocrinology* **1981; 109**:1677-82.

194. Meikle A.W., Liu X.H. and Stringham J.D. Extracellular calcium and Luteinizing hormone effects on 22-hydroxycholestrol

used for testosterone production in mouse Leydig cells. *Journal of Andrology* **1991; 12:**148-51.

195.   Clark B.J., Wells J., King S.R and Stocco D.M . The purification   Cloning and expression of a novel Luteinizing hormone induced mitochondrial protein in MA-10 mouse Leydig tumor cells. Characterization of the steriodogenic acute regulatory protein (StAR). *Journal of biological chemistry* **1994; 269**:28314-22.

196.   Lin D., Sugawara T., Strauss J.F III , Clark B.J. and Stocco D.M. Role of steroidogenic acute regulatory protein in adrenal and gonadal steroidogenesis. *Science* **1995; 267**:1828-31.

197.   Wang X.J., Liu Z., Eimerl S., Weiss A.M. and Stocco D.M. Effect of truncated forms of the steroidogenic acute regulatory protein on intramitochondrial cholesterol transfer. *Endocrinology* **1998;139**:3903-12.

198.   Omura T. and Morohashi K.   Gene regulation of steroidogenesis. *J. Steroid Biochem. Mol. Biol.* **1995;53**: 19–25.

199.   Wang X. and Stocco D.M.   The decline in testosterone biosynthesis during male aging. A consequence of multiple alteration. *Mol.Cell. Endocrinol.***2005;238**:1-7.

200.   Hauet T., Yao Z.X., Bose H.S.,Wall C.T.,Han Z.,Li W., Hales D.B., Miller W.L., Culty M., Papadopoulos V. Peripheral type benzodiazepine receptor- mediated action of steroidogenic acute regulatory protein on cholesterol entry into Leydig cell mitochondria. *Mol Endocrinol* **2005; 19(2)**:540-54.

201.   Bogan RL , Davis TL, Niswender GD. Peripheral-type benzodiazepine receptor (PBR) aggregation and absence of steroidogenic acute regulatory protein (StAR)/PBR association in

the mitochondrial membrane as determined by bioluminescence resonance energy transfer (BRET). *J Steroid Biochem Mol Biol.* **2007;104(1-2)**:61-7.

202. West, LA; Horvat, RD; Roess, DA; Barisas, BG; Juengel, JL; Niswender, GD; Steroidogenic acute regulatory protein and peripheral-type benzodiazepine receptor associate at the mitochondrial membrane. *Endocrinology* **2001;1(142)**:502-5.

203. Miller W.L. Mechanism of StAR´s regulation of mitochondrial cholesterol import. *Mol Cell Endocrinol* **2007;265-266**:46-50.

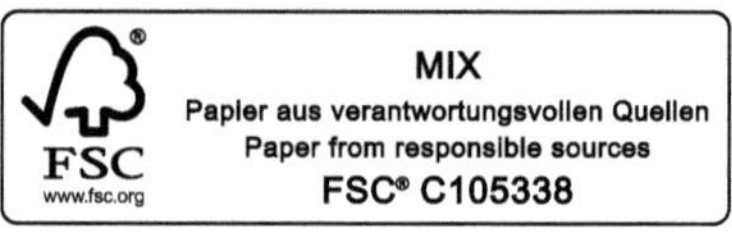

Printed by Books on Demand GmbH, Norderstedt / Germany